EXCELLER
SELECT

TOP PICKS

WOMB MATRIX

WOMB MATRIX

Decoding the sacred blueprint of womanhood

A Holistic Guide to Healing Period Problems, Balancing Hormones & Awakening Extraordinary Feminine Power

Matindra Chandra Debnath
& Katha Chakraborty

EXCELLER BOOKS®
A GLOBAL PRESS

WOMB MATRIX

Decoding the sacred blueprint of womanhood

Cover by Exceller Books

ISBN: 978-93-47397-87-5

First published in India in 2025 by Exceller Books,
An imprint of GE Group
Address: G1, Dream Apartment, Degree College Road, Belgharia,
Kolkata, 700056, India
www.excellerbooks.com

EXCELLER BOOKS®
A GLOBAL PRESS

Disclaimer

WOMB MATRIX: Decoding the Sacred Blueprint of Womanhood – A Holistic Guide to Healing Period Problems, Balancing Hormones & Awakening Extraordinary Feminine Power is intended solely for educational, informational, and inspirational purposes.

This book is not a substitute for professional medical advice, diagnosis, or treatment. The practices, ideas, and perspectives shared herein—such as womb healing, emotional clearing, natural remedies, energetic techniques, and ancestral wisdom—are drawn from holistic traditions, experiential coaching, and ancient feminine knowledge systems. While these approaches have been deeply meaningful and transformative for many, they are not intended to replace qualified medical care or evidence-based treatments offered by licensed healthcare professionals.

Always consult your physician, gynaecologist, or qualified health provider regarding any medical condition, diagnosis, or concerns, especially related to menstruation, hormonal health, fertility, menopause, or reproductive health. Never disregard or delay seeking professional advice because of something you have read in this book.

The authors, contributors, and publishers do not claim to cure, treat, or prevent any medical condition. Readers are encouraged to take personal responsibility and discernment when engaging with the content of this book. The results of holistic practices may vary depending on individual circumstances and lifestyle factors.

A Sacred Invitation

Dear Reader,

Welcome to *WOMB MATRIX: Decoding the Sacred Blueprint of Womanhood.* This book is not just a guide—it is a remembrance, a rekindling of the ancient, radiant power that lives within every woman. It is a sacred offering born from decades of deep listening—to the womb, to the Earth, and to the forgotten wisdom of our grandmothers and daughters alike.

Within these pages, you will encounter insights that bridge science and spirit, tradition and transformation, biology and mysticism. You will walk alongside stories, tools, rituals, and healing pathways that honor the sacred rhythms of the female body—your body.

This is a book for every woman who has ever felt unheard in a doctor's office, unseen in a patriarchal system, or disconnected from the divine pulse within her.

It is also for every man, parent, partner, teacher, and healer who longs to understand the mystery of womanhood with reverence and clarity.

We do not promise quick fixes or magical cures. We offer something more enduring:

A return, a reawakening, a reclamation of power that was never lost—only silenced.

Read this book

- with your heart open,
- with your mind soft,
- with your womb rooted.

✨ **Let it be a companion.**

✨ **Let it be a mirror.**

✨ **Let it be a prayer.**

Take what resonates.
Question what stirs you.
And most importantly—
Listen to yourself above all.

Because you are *divinely* guided.
You are the *matrix.*
You are the *sacred blueprint* the world has been waiting for.
With love, respect, and rising hope.

The Authors

Stories of Transformation: Real Voices from Our Healing Journey

"I initially joined the Miracle Healing Group only because of family pressure. Just a few weeks earlier, I had lost someone very close, and emotionally, I was completely shattered.

At first, I attended the classes without much presence of mind. Yet, I followed all the homework Katha Ma'am gave — and something began to shift.

What started as a routine slowly turned into a lifeline.

For years, I suffered from unbearable period pain. On those days, I would struggle just to function — school, tuitions, everything became a burden. But after joining the healing sessions and particularly the One-to-One with Ma'am, the pain started to disappear.

Today, I barely feel discomfort during my periods.

I cannot express in words how deeply grateful I am. If I hadn't said yes to this journey, I would probably still be living with that suffering. Thank you, Katha Ma'am — you are a pillar of transformation in my life."

Anwesha Mandol
College Student
Arambag

***

"My menstrual pain had become a part of me — something I thought I'd have to endure until menopause. Doctors, tests, medications — I tried them all. Nothing worked.

That's when I found Katha Chakraborty and this beautiful world of healing.

At first, I was skeptical about online healing. But through each session, I began to feel shifts I couldn't explain — only experience.

I journeyed through different types of womb healing:

Basic, Advanced, Posture-Based, Ho'oponopono, Garbha Sanskar…combined with breathwork, mudras, diet changes, yoga, and guided visualizations.

For the first time, I felt my womb being nurtured.

My pain reduced. My relationship with my body transformed.

I also experienced Akashic Healing, Mirror Healing, Inner Child Work, and Music Therapy. With every session, I became calmer, stronger, and lighter.

Today, I understand — this journey wasn't just to heal my womb. It was to heal my life.

Thank you, Katha Ma'am and Matindra Sir. You've gifted me a new way of being."

Surupa Ghosh
Homemaker
Delhi/Naihati

***

Foreword

In a world teetering between technological advancement and emotional disconnection, *Womb Matrix: Decoding the Sacred Blueprint of Womanhood* emerges as a beacon of healing, remembrance, and revolution. This is not merely a book—it is a movement, a mirror, and a manual for restoring the wisdom of the womb and honoring the cyclical nature of life itself.

Co-authored by Matindra Chandra Debnath—visionary life coach, spiritual mentor, and author of the groundbreaking book *The Constitution of the Humanity*—and Katha Chakraborty—a transformational women's life coach, healer, and menstrual health educator—this work is a brilliant confluence of **science, soul, and sacred feminine consciousness.**

For millennia, the menstrual cycle has been veiled in shame, misunderstood as a burden rather than revered as a blueprint of life. But now, as women across the globe rise to reclaim their sovereignty, *Womb Matrix* offers a timely and essential guide. It courageously dismantles taboos while gently leading the reader into a space of **healing, empowerment, and embodied wisdom.**

From the biological intricacies of the menstrual cycle to the energetics of fertility, from the trauma lodged in the womb to the path of conscious conception, this book is a **multi-dimensional journey**. It unites cutting-edge reproductive science with yogic wisdom, Ayurvedic healing, spiritual psychology, and emotional alchemy—presented in a way that is accessible, compassionate, and profoundly transformative.

This work is especially relevant in an era where PCOS, hormonal imbalances, painful periods, and infertility are silently affecting millions. Rather than offering quick fixes or temporary relief, *Womb Matrix* invites you to go deeper—into your body, into your story, and into your soul.

Whether you are:

- a young girl encountering your first bleed,
- a woman silently suffering through years of pain,
- a couple longing to conceive,
- a mother wanting to raise an empowered daughter, or
- a man wishing to understand the feminine more deeply—

This book is your sanctuary and your compass.

It is a call to remember that menstruation is not a monthly inconvenience; rather, it is a sacred pulse, a divine rhythm, a cosmic intelligence embedded in every woman.

This book also offers something larger—**a societal and spiritual invitation**. It urges humanity to awaken to the feminine principle not only as a gender identity, but as a collective necessity for healing the world. It dreams of a world where womb wisdom is taught in schools, respected in homes, honored in hospitals, and celebrated in cultures.

Womb Matrix is not just about menstrual health; it is about **rebuilding our connection to the source of life itself**.

Let this book guide you to listen to your womb, live in rhythm with your inner nature, and rise as a conscious co-creator of a healthier, more loving world.

Welcome to a new paradigm.
Welcome to the *Womb Matrix*.

With reverence and love,

Matindra Chandra Debnath
Life Coach, Visionary Edupreneur,
Author of *The Constitution of Humanity*
&
Katha Chakraborty
Women's Life Coach, Holistic Healer,
Author of *MenstruSolution*

Contents

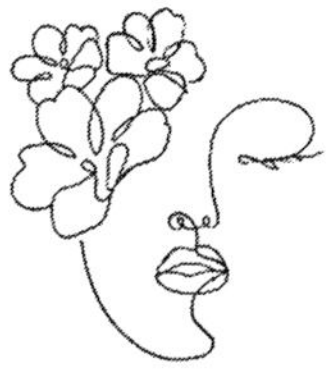

Chapter 1 | Introduction

***Womb Matrix: Decoding the Sacred Blueprint of Womanhood*: A Journey to Reclaim the Power of the Period**

"The womb is not a problem to fix; it's a universe to understand."
– Matindra Debnath

In every corner of the world, half the population bleeds cyclically—silently, discreetly, and often in shame. The monthly period, or menstruation, is perhaps one of the most misunderstood, undervalued, and culturally stigmatized biological processes in human history. Across centuries, across civilizations, and particularly in the modern World—including India—the menstrual cycle has been buried under layers of misinformation, religious taboos, gender politics, and sheer ignorance.

But what if menstruation was never meant to be a curse? What if it was the seat of your creative power, your detox process, and your body's internal moon tide guiding you into rhythm, wisdom, and rebirth every single month?

This book, *Womb Matrix: Decoding the Sacred Blueprint of Womanhood*, is a revolution in that direction — a gentle yet bold awakening, a compassionate yet scientific re-education, and a soulful reconnection to the divine intelligence of a woman's womb.

Why This Book? Why Now?

We are living in paradoxical times. On one hand, menstruation is increasingly medicalized—painkillers, hormonal pills, and period products flood the market, promising comfort without ever questioning *why* so many women today are in pain, irregular, or disconnected from their cycles.

On the other hand, a new wave of feminine awakening is rising. Women across the globe are asking deeper questions:

- Why is my cycle irregular?
- Why do I have painful cramps?
- Why was I never taught to honor my bleeding days?
- What is my womb really trying to tell me?

This book was born from that space of inquiry, of deep listening to the cries and whispers of the womb. It is the result of many years of coaching and healing girls and women struggling with irregular period, painful period, heavy flow, spotting, excessively longer period, PCOS, PCOD, endometriosis, adenomyosis, infertility, emotional trauma, and spiritual disconnection from their feminine essence.

Womb Matrix: Decoding the Sacred Blueprint of Womanhood is more than a book. It is a reclamation, a healing journey, a guide to transform your period from a problem into a portal.

What Lies Ahead in These Pages?

In these chapters, you will not find just theories or textbook explanations. You will find stories, science, spirituality, and embodied wisdom drawn from Ayurveda, Yogic practices, Tantra, ancient menstrual customs, and modern neuroscience.

We will explore:

- The biological brilliance of the menstrual cycle.
- The connection between menstruation and the Moon.
- Ayurvedic and yogic views on menstruation as a time of purification.
- The importance of menstrual rest and the ancient practice of *Rajaswala Paricharya.*

- The cultural distortions that have made periods "impure" in the eyes of society.
- The subconscious programming girls receive about shame, silence, and survival.
- The relationship between period problems and unresolved emotional trauma.
- Fertility awareness, hormonal balance, and the wisdom of conscious conception.
- Tools like womb healing, forgiveness, gratitude practices, and breathwork to reconnect with your body's wisdom.

Each chapter ends not just with reflection, but with actionable healing rituals—simple yet powerful practices that will help you shift your relationship with your cycle.

Why Are Menstruators in Pain Today?

Today's girls are getting their first period not with celebration but with confusion. Painkillers are being normalized at age 13. Girls are taught to hide pads up their sleeves, avoid temples, pretend nothing is happening, and keep performing at school or work regardless of what their body is going through. At the root of these experiences lies **deep energetic disconnection**.

Modern women are taught to operate within a masculine, linear, productive framework. The menstrual cycle, however, is cyclical. It needs rhythm, slowness, rest, and renewal. When women suppress these natural needs month after month, year after year, it leads to symptoms: irregularity, PCOD, endometriosis, infertility, and burnout.

So the pain is not just physical. It is **cultural, emotional, and energetic**. And yet, every pain is a signal—a message from the womb, asking you to return home to yourself.

The Forgotten Power of the Period

Ancient texts like the **Garbha Upanishad** and Ayurvedic scriptures revered the womb and menstrual blood as sacred.

Women were seen as creators of life and carriers of divine Shakti. In tribal and indigenous cultures, menstruation was not dirty but divine. Women would retreat into Red Tents or Moon Lodges to rest, dream, receive visions, and regenerate their bodies.

In contrast, today's girls are rushed, ridiculed, or neglected. They have no menstrual education beyond biology textbooks, which are at best vague knowledge, no emotional holding, and no feminine mentorship.

This book attempts to change that. It is my offering to every girl and woman who has ever felt ashamed of her cycle, hated her body, or questioned her worth. It is also a wake-up call for mothers, teachers, healers, and policy-makers to co-create a world where menstruation is honored, supported, and celebrated.

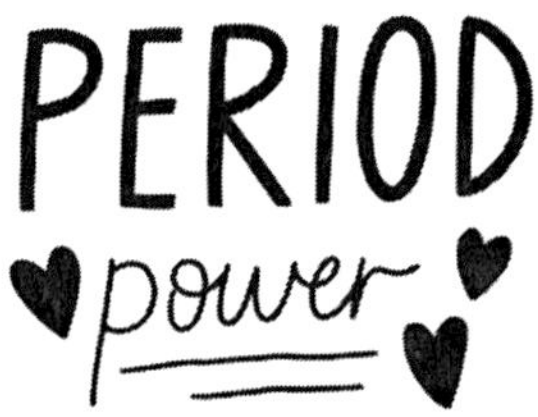

Healing Begins with Awareness

Healing your cycle does not require expensive pills or endless doctor visits. It begins with awareness, with listening, with deep curiosity and with a willingness to see your period not as a monthly problem, but as a monthly message.

Womb Matrix: Decoding the Sacred Blueprint of Womanhood offers you a way to decode that message.

The path is layered. First, you'll learn to observe, then, to accept, then, to realign, and ultimately, to embody the wisdom of your cyclical nature. That's where your real feminine power lives—not in being consistent, but in being connected.

A Personal Note to You, Dear Reader

I wrote this book not as an expert speaking to the masses, but as a woman who walked this path herself. I have bled with pain. I have cried into the silence of my womb. I have asked why the world does not see the sacredness of menstruation.

But I have also seen miracles, women who regulated their cycles with womb healing, couples who conceived after years of "unexplained infertility", girls who went from hating their periods to waiting for them with love and pride.

I invite you to read this book with an open heart and a soft belly. Let the stories, insights, and practices move through your body. Let them reawaken what you already know, deep inside:

Your body is not broken.
Your period is not a punishment.
Your womb holds the map to your healing.

Welcome to *Womb Matrix:*
Decoding the Sacred Blueprint of Womanhood
Let's walk back to the source—together.

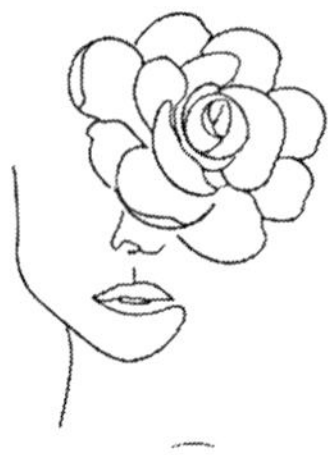

Chapter 2 | The Biology of Menstruation — Anatomy and Physiology of the Female Reproductive System

Menstruation is a natural, cyclical biological process fundamental to human reproduction. It is a visible manifestation of a highly complex system that regulates fertility, hormone balance, and reproductive health in women. To truly understand menstruation, one must explore the anatomy of the female reproductive system, the hormonal interplay, and the phases of the menstrual cycle.

Anatomy of the Female Reproductive System

The female reproductive system comprises both external and internal organs, each playing specific roles in menstruation and reproduction.

External Genitalia

- **Vulva:** The external part of the female genitalia, including the mons pubis, labia majora and minora, clitoris, urethral opening, and vaginal opening.
- **Vagina:** A muscular, elastic canal extending from the vulva to the cervix, serving as the birth canal and the passage for menstrual flow.

Internal Organs

- **Ovaries:** Two almond-shaped organs located on either side of the uterus. The ovaries produce eggs (ova) and secrete hormones such as estrogen and progesterone that regulate the menstrual cycle.
- **Fallopian Tubes (Oviducts):** Tubes extending from each ovary to the uterus. They transport the ovulated egg to the uterus and are the usual site of fertilization.
- **Uterus:** A hollow, muscular, pear-shaped organ. The uterus has three layers:
    - **Endometrium:** The inner mucosal lining that thickens in preparation for possible pregnancy and sheds during menstruation if fertilization does not occur.
    - **Myometrium:** The thick, muscular middle layer responsible for uterine contractions during menstruation and childbirth.
    - **Perimetrium:** The outer serous layer covering the uterus.
- **Cervix:** The lower, narrow part of the uterus opening into the vagina, producing cervical mucus which changes in consistency during the cycle to facilitate or prevent sperm passage.

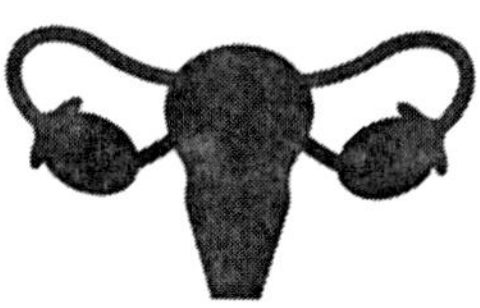

The Menstrual Cycle: Phases and Hormonal Control

The menstrual cycle is an orchestrated sequence of events regulated primarily by hormones produced by the hypothalamus, pituitary gland, and ovaries. It typically lasts about 28 days, though 21-35 days is considered normal.

Key Hormones

- **Gonadotropin-releasing hormone (GnRH):** Released by the hypothalamus, stimulates the pituitary to secrete FSH and LH.
- **Follicle-stimulating hormone (FSH):** Stimulates ovarian follicles to mature eggs.
- **Luteinizing hormone (LH):** Triggers ovulation and corpus luteum formation.
- **Estrogen:** Produced by growing follicles, thickens the endometrium and regulates other cycle components.
- **Progesterone:** Secreted by the corpus luteum post-ovulation, stabilizes and maintains the endometrium.

Phases of the Menstrual Cycle

- Menstrual Phase (Days 1–5)
  - The cycle begins with menstruation, the shedding of the functional layer of the endometrium when fertilization does not occur.
  - Menstrual bleeding lasts 3 to 7 days on average and is composed of blood, tissue debris, mucus, and vaginal secretions.
- Follicular (Proliferative) Phase (Days 1–13)
  - FSH stimulates several ovarian follicles to mature; one dominant follicle continues to develop.
  - The maturing follicle produces estrogen, which promotes thickening (proliferation) of the endometrial lining, preparing the uterus for a potential embryo.
  - Estrogen also causes cervical mucus to become thin and watery, facilitating sperm movement.
- Ovulation (Day 14)
  - A surge in LH from the pituitary triggers ovulation—the release of a mature egg from the dominant follicle into the fallopian tube.
  - The egg survives about 12-24 hours if not fertilized.

- Luteal (Secretory) Phase (Days 15–28)
  - The ruptured follicle transforms into the corpus luteum, secreting progesterone (and some estrogen).
  - Progesterone causes the endometrium to become thick, glandular, and rich in blood vessels, optimizing it for implantation.
  - If fertilization does not occur, the corpus luteum degenerates, leading to a drop in progesterone and estrogen, triggering the next menstruation.

Menstruation: The Shedding Process

- The decline in progesterone causes blood vessels in the endometrium to constrict, leading to ischemia (loss of oxygen).
- This ischemia causes the upper layers of the endometrium to break down and detach.
- Enzymes digest the tissue, and contractions of the myometrium help expel the tissue and blood through the cervix and vagina.
- Menstrual flow consists of blood, endometrial cells, mucus, and vaginal secretions.

The Ovarian Cycle and Follicular Development

- At birth, females have approximately 1-2 million primordial follicles; by puberty, about 300,000 remain.
- Each menstrual cycle, about 5-20 follicles begin maturation, but only one reaches full maturity.
- The mature follicle contains the oocyte, which will be released during ovulation.

The Endocrine Feedback Loop

- The menstrual cycle is regulated by a feedback loop involving the hypothalamus, pituitary gland, and ovaries.

- Rising estrogen levels initially inhibit FSH to ensure only one follicle matures, but then stimulate the LH surge, causing ovulation.
- After ovulation, progesterone and estrogen from the corpus luteum inhibit GnRH, FSH, and LH secretion to prevent further ovulation during the same cycle.

Common Biological Variations and Menstrual Health

- Cycle length and flow can vary among individuals and within a person's lifetime.
- Factors like stress, nutrition, illness, and hormonal imbalances can affect cycle regularity.
- Disorders such as amenorrhea (absence of menstruation), dysmenorrhea (painful menstruation), menorrhagia (heavy bleeding), and oligomenorrhea (infrequent menstruation) arise from disruptions in this delicate system.

Conclusion

The menstrual cycle is an elegant, finely tuned biological rhythm that orchestrates fertility and reproductive health. Its processes—from hormone signaling to the structural changes in the ovaries and uterus—represent a remarkable example of human physiology and evolutionary adaptation. Understanding this biology is the foundation for empowering women with knowledge, helping dispel myths and taboos, and supporting holistic health.

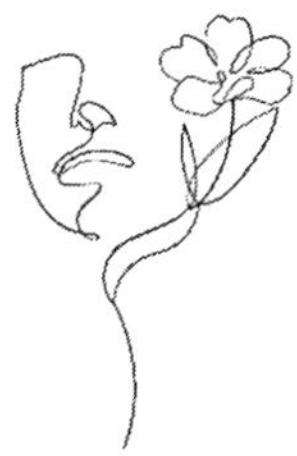

Chapter 3 | Ancestral Wounds and Societal Shame around Menstruation and Fertility from Silence to Sacred Power

"You don't just inherit eye color or height from your ancestors—
You inherit their silence, their shame, and their unhealed pain too."

The Invisible Thread of Pain

Menstruation and fertility are not just physical events. They are energetic, emotional, and ancestral experiences woven into the very fabric of womanhood. For millennia, this sacred biological rhythm has been subjected to shame, silence, suppression, and distortion—so much so that most women today cannot speak about their periods or reproductive struggles without feeling discomfort or judgment.

This discomfort is not accidental; it is inherited, ancestral, and cultural. And unless we choose to name it, feel it, and release it, it continues to shape our present.

As a woman begins to explore her cycle, she often finds herself encountering not just her personal pain, but echoes of her mother's grief, her grandmother's silence, and the collective wounds of countless women before her.

This is the hidden layer of menstruation and fertility: the ancestral wound.

What Are Ancestral Wounds?

Ancestral wounds are unresolved emotional imprints passed down through generations. These wounds are not always spoken about openly. In many families, especially in traditional societies, sensitive topics like miscarriage, infertility, abuse, or reproductive loss are buried in silence.

But what remains unspoken does not disappear.

It seeps into the DNA. It travels through the womb-line. It sits in the cells of daughters and granddaughters as inexplicable sadness, confusion, shame, or fear.

Ancestral wounds are more than memories. They are emotional legacies.

Imagine a young woman who never knew that her grandmother was forced into child marriage, had five miscarriages, or lived with the pain of being called "barren." That grandmother may have never shared her story—but her suffering lives on in the granddaughter's womb, silently influencing how she relates to her own cycle, her body, her self-worth.

The Shame That Was Inherited

There was a time in ancient India, and in many indigenous cultures, when menstruating women were seen as sacred. Their blood was a symbol of life, their bodies were temples of wisdom, and their wombs were portals of divine creation.

But with the rise of patriarchy and institutionalized religion, this perception changed. A woman's body began to be viewed as dangerous, impure, and in need of control. New myths and restrictions were created to suppress her power, especially the mysterious and powerful phenomena of menstruation and reproduction.

Over time, these beliefs became normalized:

- Menstruating women are impure.
- Women should not enter temples, kitchens, or sacred spaces during their period.
- Girls must hide their pads and their pain.

- Infertility is a personal failure or divine punishment.
- Talking about miscarriage, sexual trauma, or womb pain is taboo.

This collective shame turned natural biological processes into subjects of fear, disgust, and silence. And that silence became a disease passed from generation to generation.

From Puberty to Pain: How Shame Is Learned

The transmission of menstrual shame begins early. Most girls receive no real education about their menstrual cycle—only a hurried explanation, often laced with fear or awkwardness. They are told:

- "Don't talk about this in front of boys."
- "You're dirty during these days."
- "Be careful, or you'll get pregnant."
- "Stay away from sacred spaces."

Rarely is a girl told, "Your body is entering a sacred cycle. This blood is not a curse; it is a blessing. This pain is not punishment; it is purification. You are not less during your period—you are more."

So the girl internalizes her first bleed as a moment of shame, confusion, or burden. She hides her pain; she hides her pad; she hides her power. And thus begins a lifelong disconnect between her and her womb.

The Silent Struggles of Our Mothers

Many of our mothers, grandmothers, and great-grandmothers bore children in environments of silence, pressure, and pain. They often experienced:

- The trauma of repeated miscarriages without emotional support
- Being blamed or abandoned for infertility
- Coerced abortions or gender-based violence
- Emotional abuse during pregnancy
- Isolation during menstruation

And yet, they never spoke of it.

Not because it did not hurt—but because there was no space to speak, no permission to grieve, no culture that honored their pain.

But trauma does not end when it is ignored; rather, it buries itself deeper into the womb, into the lineage, into the subconscious. This is the essence of *epigenetics*—the science of how emotional wounds become biological memories.

How Womb Shame Affects Fertility

When a woman desires to conceive, her womb becomes more than just an organ. It becomes a field of energy, memory, and emotion. It holds not only her reproductive capacity—but also her beliefs, her fears, and her ancestral inheritance.

If her womb is holding shame from past generations, trauma from her own life, or rejection of her feminine essence, this creates subtle but powerful blocks to conception.

- She may experience irregular cycles, PCOD, and endometriosis
- She may find herself unable to relax into intimacy or pleasure
- She may carry subconscious beliefs like "I'm not good enough to be a mother" or "My body is broken"

These beliefs can manifest as real, diagnosable conditions—but at the root, there is often a deeper, invisible pain: a womb that has not been heard, honored, or healed.

Breaking the Cycle: From Wound to Wisdom

The first step to healing is awareness. We cannot change what we do not name. We cannot heal what we do not feel.

As women, we must start by acknowledging the lineage we come from—not with blame, but with compassion. Our mothers and grandmothers did the best they could in the environments they were born into. But now, we have the tools, the voice, and the support to do things differently.

We can begin to:

- Talk about our cycles without shame
- Learn the spiritual and biological truths of menstruation
- Hold space for others to share their womb stories
- Heal our ancestral wounds through practices like womb healing, breathwork, journaling, and forgiveness
- Celebrate our periods as sacred thresholds, not medical problems

This chapter, dear reader, is an invitation to begin that journey.

A New Legacy Begins with You

The shame that was passed down for generations ends with you.
The silence that muted your grandmother's pain ends with you.
The guilt, the fear, the hiding, all end with you.
You are not just healing your own body.
You are healing an entire bloodline.
You are creating a new story for the girls yet to bleed.
Let this chapter be the moment you turn inward—not with judgment, but with love.
Sit with your womb, breathe into her, and ask her what she needs. Listen.
She is not your enemy. She is your oldest friend.

Welcome to the first step of MenstruSolution—
Not a book, but a return to your sacred rhythm.
Not just a solution, but a reclamation.
Let the healing begin.

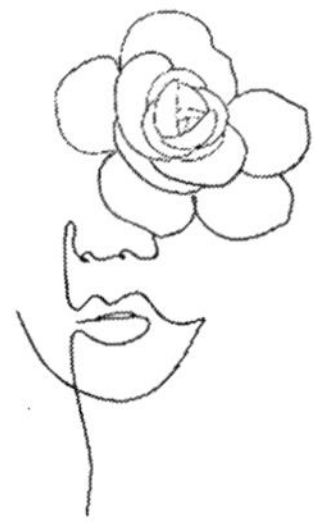

Chapter 4|The Path to Liberation: Shifting Consciousness and Holistic Healing

"The womb is not just a place of conception. It is the origin of power, the gateway to intuition, and the sacred seat of feminine wisdom."

To step out of the inherited legacy of shame, ancestral wounds, and silence around menstruation and fertility, women must embark on a path of deep awareness, loving acceptance, and holistic healing. This chapter serves as a compass, pointing toward liberation. It offers a powerful vision: menstruation is not a curse to be concealed but a sacred rhythm to be honored. And that every woman, regardless of age, history, or struggle, can awaken her womb wisdom.

Awareness: Redefining the Narrative

The first step is awareness—the conscious act of seeing menstruation and fertility through a new, empowered lens.

- **Menstruation is not impure.** It is a time of spiritual rest, a monthly reset gifted by nature.
- **Reproductive power is not a burden.** It is a divine blessing that allows for the creation and nurturing of life.

We must shed the limiting definitions imposed by society and reclaim the truth that has always been ours: menstruation is a sacred, biological, emotional, and energetic experience.

Open Conversation: Breaking the Silence

Healing begins with voice. For generations, menstruation and fertility were surrounded by silence—even among mothers and daughters.

Let us create a new culture:

- Where mothers speak openly with their daughters
- Where stories of miscarriage, conception, infertility, and healing are shared with dignity, not shame
- Where young girls learn to honor their bodies, instead of hiding them

When we speak, we pass down not just stories but strength.

Healing and Forgiveness: Returning Home to the Womb

Healing is not about fixing a broken body; it is about restoring a whole person. It is about remembering what has been forgotten.

- Repair the relationship with your own body
- Forgive your ancestors for the silence and pain they carried
- Reclaim the maternal power that lives within you

When a woman reconnects with her womb—not just as an organ, but as an energy center—she begins to experience inner rebirth. This is the essence of womb healing.

The Sacred Truth of Menstruation and Reproduction

Society has veiled the truth about menstruation with layers of cultural taboos and restrictions. But when stripped of these illusions, what remains is powerful:

- **Menstruation is a sacred force.**
- **Reproduction is a spiritual journey.**

Today's woman has the power to step beyond the inherited limitations and create a new story—a story of confidence, reverence, and love.

Understanding the Menstrual Cycle as a Spiritual and Detox Journey

The menstrual cycle is not just a physical event—it is a spiritual detox. Every month, a woman's body initiates a process of cleansing, renewal, and energetic alignment. Let us look deeper.

- The womb naturally releases old blood and toxins.
- This physical release is also emotional and energetic. Women often feel anger, grief, or past emotions surface during this time.
- Intuition is heightened. The inner voice becomes clearer—helping us recognize what needs to be released and what needs to be embraced.

Period means Pause.

Pause to rest. Pause to reflect. Pause to listen.

Ask yourself:

- ➢ What is my body saying?
- ➢ What emotions are rising?
- ➢ What do I need to let go of?

The Womb as a Sacred Energy Center

The womb is not just a biological structure. In ancient wisdom systems, it is the seat of the **Sacral Chakra** —the center of creation, sensuality, and feminine energy. Each cycle

- Releases old memories and energetic imprints
- Clears emotional residues
- Prepares to receive new creative energy

Just as a river cleans its path, the womb maintains the purity of the life-giving channel. Menstruation is a sacred reset.

Period Self-Care = Self-Love

To care for yourself during your period is not indulgence. It is reverence. The body and mind need:

- Warmth (e.g. warm water or heating pads)
- Sattvic, easily digestible foods
- Gentle yoga or movement
- Emotional tenderness

Treating yourself with love and respect during your period signals to your subconscious that your cycle is sacred, not shameful.

The Menstrual Cycle as a Fulfilment Cycle: Creation, Destruction, Rebirth

Each month, a woman undergoes a sacred transformation that mirrors the cycle of life itself. This rhythm contains four powerful phases:

- **Menstrual Phase (Day 1–5)**
    - **Theme:** Release & Rest
    - **Gift:** Letting go of physical and emotional toxins
    - **Practices:**
        - ✓ Rest in solitude
        - ✓ Journal, meditate
        - ✓ Practice gentle breathwork

This is your winter. Trust the stillness.

- **Follicular Phase (Day 6–13)**
    - **Theme:** Creativity, New Beginnings
    - **Gift:** Clarity, inspiration, motivation
    - **Practices:**
        - ✓ Begin new projects
        - ✓ Set intentions
        - ✓ Take action on dreams

This is your spring. Energy is rising.

- **Ovulation Phase (Day 14–17)**
    - **Theme:** Magnetism, Expression, Connection
    - **Gift:** High energy, social vitality, beauty

  - **Practices:**
    - ✓ Spend time with loved ones
    - ✓ Express yourself creatively
    - ✓ Practice gratitude and joy

This is your summer. Shine full.

- **Luteal Phase (Day 18–28)**
  - **Theme:** Introspection, Boundaries, Preparation
  - **Gift:** Inner clarity, shadow work, sacred boundaries
  - **Practices:**
    - ✓ Say no to what drains you
    - ✓ Practice self-reflection
    - ✓ Prepare for emotional release

This is your autumn. Go inward.

Reclaiming the Wisdom of the Cycle

Your menstrual cycle is not a monthly inconvenience. It is:

- A natural detox for the body
- A purification of the mind
- A reconnection with the soul
- A cycle of renewal, creativity, and transformation

It teaches you how to:

- Rest without guilt
- Listen deeply to your intuition
- Nurture your dreams in alignment with nature

Every month, you are given a blueprint to recreate your life, heal your past, and move forward with power.

Final Reflections

Menstruation is not just bleeding. It is an initiation, a ceremony, a sacred pause that invites you to release what no longer serves you and prepare for what is to come.

Let us no longer treat our cycles as medical events to be hidden or managed. Let us treat them as sacred rhythms to be honored.

Welcome to a new way of living—one that honors the womb, celebrates the period, and reclaims the power of womanhood.

This is the essence of MenstruSolution.

Let the healing continue.

Chapter 5 | The Silent Epidemic: Menstrual Problems Faced by Modern Women and Girls

Despite medical progress and greater awareness, menstrual health remains one of the most neglected areas of women's wellness. Millions of girls, women, and even mothers suffer silently each month—often believing that pain, irregularity, or emotional turmoil during menstruation is just "normal."

But in truth, these signs point to deeper imbalances that the body is trying to communicate. Menstruation is a vital barometer of a woman's overall physical, emotional, and spiritual health. When the cycle is off balance, it is not just a reproductive issue—it is a call for holistic healing.

The Menstrual Struggles of Teenagers: The First Alarm Bells

- **Irregular Periods after Menarche:** It is common for adolescent girls to experience irregular periods for the first 1–2 years after their first bleed. But when this irregularity persists, it becomes a warning signal. Contributing factors include:
  - Hormonal imbalance during puberty
  - Poor diet (junk food, sugar, processed snacks)
  - Inadequate sleep and overuse of screens

   - Excessive mental stress (academic, social, emotional)
- **Painful Periods (Primary Dysmenorrhea):** Many teenage girls suffer from severe cramps that are often ignored or dismissed. For some, it becomes so unbearable that they miss school, avoid sports, and withdraw socially. In most cases, this is due to spasms in the uterus, but in some cases, it may be an early sign of conditions like endometriosis.
- **Heavy Bleeding (Menorrhagia):** Excessive menstrual bleeding in adolescents is not only exhausting but may lead to anemia, fatigue, low immunity, and low self-esteem. This must not be ignored.
- **Absent or Very Light Periods (Amenorrhea):** This is particularly seen in girls under emotional distress, those who are underweight, or those who over-exercise or diet. It is a serious indication of a disrupted reproductive system.
- **PCOS Symptoms in Teens:** Increasingly, young girls are showing early signs of PCOS:
   - Irregular periods
   - Acne and oily skin
   - Hair fall or facial hair growth
   - Weight gain

These symptoms must be addressed early to prevent long-term complications.

- **Emotional Changes: PMS, Anxiety & Depression:** Premenstrual Syndrome (PMS) starts appearing during teenage years. Without proper support, it often develops into anxiety disorders, mood imbalances, or chronic stress.

Menstrual Problems in Young and Married Women: The Crisis Deepens

- **Polycystic Ovary Syndrome (PCOS):** One of the most common disorders today, affecting 4 out of 10 women. Caused by insulin resistance and hormonal imbalance. PCOS leads to:
    - Irregular or absent periods
    - Facial hair, acne, weight gain
    - Difficulty in conceiving
- **Fibroids and Cysts:** Benign growths in the uterus often go undiagnosed. Symptoms include:
    - Heavy menstrual bleeding
    - Pelvic pain
    - Bloating or constipation
    - Fertility issues
- **Irregular Cycles and Hormonal Chaos:** Urban lifestyle, career stress, gadget overuse, and poor sleep hygiene disrupt endocrine harmony, resulting in:
    - Unpredictable periods
    - Painful ovulation
    - Hormonal migraines
- **Infertility and Recurrent Miscarriages:** Chronic menstrual disturbances—if ignored—lead to subfertility. Repeated miscarriages, implantation failure, and conception difficulty often have roots in untreated menstrual problems.

Menstrual Concerns in Midlife and Perimenopause

- **Irregular or Skipped Periods:** After age 40, the menstrual cycle becomes erratic. But sudden disappearance or extremely painful cycles may signal premature ovarian failure or deep hormonal deficiency.
- **Hot Flashes, Mood Swings, Insomnia:** These are not just menopausal clichés. Estrogen withdrawal affects the nervous system, leading to:

    - Night sweats
    - Emotional vulnerability
    - Loss of libido
    - Sleep disturbances
- **Bone Health and Menstrual Cessation:** Post-menstrual life brings with it the risk of osteoporosis, joint pain, and fragile bones due to declining estrogen.
- **Changes in Beauty and Vitality:** Thinning hair, dry skin, and premature aging are visible symptoms of internal hormonal decline.

Beyond Biology: The Hidden Roots of Menstrual Suffering

Despite high-tech scans and pharmaceutical treatments, many menstrual problems persist because we have been treating the symptom, not the source.

Modern medicine rarely considers this:

"The womb is not just a physical organ—it is a sacred memory center."

Deep in our cellular memory, unprocessed emotions, ancestral trauma, and societal shame lodge themselves within the womb. Pain, infertility, or erratic cycles are the body's cries for emotional and spiritual attention.

This is where metaphysics and energy medicine come in.

What Truly Causes Menstrual Problems?

- **Hormonal Imbalance:** The most immediate cause of period-related issues. The delicate dance of estrogen, progesterone, LH, and FSH gets disrupted by:
    - Processed food and sugar
    - Blue light exposure at night
    - Lack of sleep
    - Chronic stress
    - Sedentary lifestyle
- **Emotional Suppression & Stress:** Stress activates cortisol, which suppresses reproductive hormones.

Emotional stress, heartbreak, people-pleasing, and lack of boundaries all impact the womb directly.

- **Nutritional Deficiency & Lifestyle Errors:** When women skip meals, consume excess caffeine, or follow social media diets, they starve their womb of nutrients like Iron, B12, Zinc, and Magnesium—all vital for hormone production.
- **Weight Fluctuations**
  - Excess fat stores estrogen, creating hormonal havoc.
  - Underweight women may stop menstruating entirely.

Both extremes disturb ovulation and menstrual harmony.

- **Repressed Emotions & Ancestral Wounds:** Women carry generations of silence, shame, and sacrifice in their bloodlines. This gets embedded into the womb space, manifesting as disease.

The Urgency of Healing: A Womb Call to Action

Menstrual disorders are not punishments—they are wake-up calls.

They ask us to:

- Reclaim our rhythms
- Nourish our body with love
- Allow emotional release
- Honor our womb as a source of wisdom

No pill can heal shame. No scan can detect generational pain. Only self-awareness, Womb Healing, and feminine wisdom can do that.

As you journey deeper into this book, you will discover how to align your cycle with nature, clear trauma from your womb space, and step into your feminine power fully.

This is not just about managing symptoms. It is about rising in sacred remembrance.

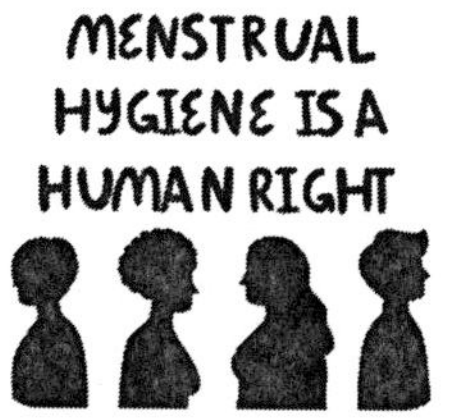

Menstruation is not a medical event—it is a mystical portal. Let us treat it as such. Let us begin the healing. Let us answer the call of the Womb.

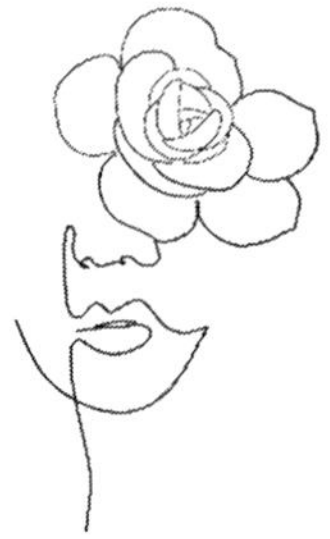

Chapter 6 | When the Body Speaks: Consequences of Ignoring Menstrual Health

A woman's menstrual cycle is not just a biological function; it is a vital indicator of her overall health. Just as a tree shows signs when its roots are unhealthy, the female body offers powerful signals when something is off-balance. Yet too often, menstrual irregularities and symptoms are ignored or dismissed as "normal," when in fact they are red flags from the body — calling out for attention, care, and correction.

In this chapter, we explore the dangerous consequences of ignoring menstrual problems and how something seemingly small today can cascade into serious physical, emotional, and even spiritual consequences over time.

Infertility: The Silent Aftermath

Unresolved menstrual irregularities and hormonal imbalances are among the leading causes of infertility today. When a woman's cycles are erratic, overly painful, or missing entirely, it reflects internal disharmony that can interfere with ovulation, egg quality, and the uterine environment required for conception.

The tragedy is that many women only begin to investigate these issues seriously when they are ready to conceive, often discovering too late that deep-rooted problems had been silently progressing for years.

Your menstrual health is your fertility health. Timely care can make the difference between a joyful conception journey and years of struggle.

Miscarriage: When the Body Cannot Hold

A weakened or imbalanced reproductive system may struggle to support a growing pregnancy. Hormonal insufficiency, uterine conditions, and chronic stress can all compromise the delicate environment needed to sustain life.

Unresolved menstrual issues make the womb less resilient, and this vulnerability may manifest in repeated miscarriages, leading to deep emotional trauma and physical exhaustion.

Healing menstrual disorders early can fortify the womb's strength and prevent future loss.

The Mental Health Spiral: Depression, Anxiety, and Beyond

Women with long-standing menstrual issues often find themselves battling mood swings, irritability, anxiety, and chronic sadness. This is not just hormonal — it is also the emotional weight of living in a body that feels out of sync.

Unaddressed menstrual distress can spiral into:

- Chronic depression
- Panic attacks
- Body image issues
- Emotional burnout

Mental health is deeply tied to hormonal rhythms. If those rhythms are disturbed, the mind and soul suffer too.

Physical Weakness, Fatigue, and Anemia

Heavy bleeding, especially when left untreated, can lead to iron deficiency or anaemia. This not only causes fatigue but also weakens the immune system, diminishes cognitive performance, and affects quality of life.

Women with undiagnosed or untreated menorrhagia often feel:

- Perpetually tired
- Dizzy or short of breath
- Unable to concentrate or engage fully in life

Without proper care, this becomes a chronic condition that dims a woman's energy, vitality, and zest for life.

Chronic Diseases: Heart Issues and Diabetes

Modern medical research has confirmed that prolonged hormonal imbalance increases the risk of cardiovascular problems and metabolic disorders like diabetes.

Estrogen and progesterone do far more than regulate the cycle. They influence heart health, glucose metabolism, and inflammation levels. When these hormones are imbalanced, the entire endocrine system suffers.

Ignoring menstrual health is not just a reproductive risk; it's a total health risk.

Osteoporosis: The Hidden Cost of Hormonal Decline

As estrogen levels decline — particularly in untreated menstrual or menopausal imbalances — bone density occurs. Osteoporosis is a silent disease that often reveals itself only after fractures or irreversible damage.

Preventative menstrual health is the key to preventing the early onset of this debilitating condition.

The Web of Daily Stress: Its Hidden Role in Menstrual Chaos

- ***The Body under Siege***

From morning deadlines to evening responsibilities, stress weaves through every woman's life. While some level of stress is unavoidable, chronic, unrelenting pressure alters the body's hormonal environment in harmful ways.

Cortisol, the primary stress hormone, is a major disruptor. Elevated cortisol affects the **Hypothalamus-Pituitary-Ovarian (HPO) Axis**, which governs menstruation. When this axis is compromised, cycles become erratic, ovulation may cease, and PMS symptoms intensify.

- ***Scientific Findings on Stress and Menstruation***

Studies have repeatedly shown that high stress levels are linked to:

- Irregular menstruation
- Anovulation (failure to release eggs)
- Severe PMS and PMDD
- Dysmenorrhea (painful periods)

This makes emotional wellness, mindfulness, and stress reduction not luxuries but **medical necessities** for a healthy cycle.

- ***Diet, Lifestyle, and Menstrual Health***

Processed Foods and Hormonal Chaos

The rise of fast food, packaged snacks, and chemically preserved items has paralleled a sharp increase in menstrual complaints. These foods:

- Contain trans fats and synthetic chemicals
- Disrupt hormonal signaling
- Increase bodily inflammation

Result: Heavier, more painful, and irregular periods.

- ***Hydration: The Forgotten Medicine***

Insufficient water intake impairs blood circulation and lymphatic drainage, contributing to menstrual cramps, bloating, and toxin accumulation.

Your womb, like every organ, thrives on hydration.

The Sleep Crisis

Blue light exposure, late-night screen use, and insomnia reduce **melatonin** and **growth hormone** production. Both are essential for hormonal regulation and restorative repair.

Inadequate sleep equals:

- Hormonal misfiring
- Weakened immunity
- Aggravated menstrual pain

Movement is Medicine

A sedentary lifestyle is one of the least-discussed but most damaging contributors to menstrual disharmony. Physical movement improves blood flow, balances hormones, reduces stress, and promotes endorphin release.

Regular yoga, dance, walking, or any joyful movement can transform a woman's cycle from painful to powerful.

Hormonal Imbalance: The Root Cause of All Menstrual Disorders

- ***Thyroid Dysfunctions***

The thyroid regulates metabolism and interacts closely with reproductive hormones. Hypothyroidism or hyperthyroidism can cause:

  - Missed periods
  - Excessive bleeding
  - Infertility

- **Insulin Resistance and PCOS**

In Polycystic Ovary Syndrome (PCOS), insulin resistance disrupts ovarian function, leading to irregular cycles, acne, hirsutism, and weight gain.

- **Estrogen Dominance**

Excess estrogen can suppress progesterone, resulting in heavy bleeding, mood swings, and increased risk of fibroids or endometriosis.

Hormonal health is a delicate symphony. When one note is off, the whole rhythm is disrupted.

What Happens If Menstrual Problems Remain Unresolved?

- Long-term reproductive damage (infertility, miscarriage)
- Chronic physical health issues (anemia, osteoporosis, diabetes)
- Mental health degradation (depression, anxiety, fatigue)
- Reduced quality of life (pain, low energy, poor focus)
- Disconnection from body and feminine energy (loss of intuition, shame, lack of self-love)

Listen to the Whispers Before They Become Screams

Every menstrual symptom is your body speaking to you. Whether it is pain, irregularity, or mood change, it is not just a monthly inconvenience. It is a **message,** a call to awareness, a request for healing.

Let us begin to listen. Let us care enough to respond.
Because menstrual health is not just about periods.
It is about the quality of a woman's entire life.

Chapter 7 | The Only Path Is Healing: From Pain to Power

In today's fast-paced world, women are expected to be everything to everyone. Mothers are juggling home, work, children, in-laws, and often even elderly parents. Meanwhile, young women and students are immersed in exams, ambitions, and the invisible burden of proving themselves worthy.

In this relentless race, one thing often gets left behind: **the self**. And most tragically, the cries of the body—its whispers, then its shouts—go unheard.

The Invisible Cry of the Feminine Body

Your body does not forget. When your body is ignored, neglected, or silenced, it speaks louder.

The sharp pain before your period, the fatigue that won't go away, the sudden mood swings, the cycle that keeps shifting, the weight gain, and the anxiety — all of it is your body speaking to you in the only language it knows.

And when we do not listen, that language becomes louder, more painful, and more complicated—sometimes leading to infertility, miscarriage, deep depression, chronic fatigue, and hormonal disorders.

But here is the **hopeful truth**:

No Matter the Problem, Healing Is Always Possible

Not through pills, not by running away, but by **turning inward,** by learning the sacred language of your body, by choosing to heal.

What is Healing?

Healing is not just the absence of illness. It is the return to wholeness. It is the conscious act of reconnecting to your body, mind, and soul. Healing means listening to your inner wounds, releasing suppressed emotions, balancing your hormones, and rebuilding your relationship with your femininity.

Healing is not magic, but it is miraculous. It is a sacred, step-by-step inner journey back to your truth.

Why is Healing the Only Real Solution?

Because menstrual issues are never just physical, they are messages.

Hormones are not isolated chemicals; they are deeply influenced by your thoughts, emotions, and the signals sent by your **nervous system**.

You may be eating the healthiest food and doing regular workouts, but if you are still holding onto unresolved grief, anger, guilt, or a feeling of unworthiness, your hormones will remain imbalanced.

Healing Is the Only Path That Goes to the Root

It releases the silent pain stored in your womb. It clears the emotional fog clouding your mind. It teaches you to love your body again.

How Healing Transforms Your Menstrual Health

- *Emotional Clearing:* Many of us carry childhood trauma, family conflicts, and unspoken emotional wounds that stay trapped in the body. Unless they are released, the body cannot heal. Healing allows you to shed those burdens.

- *Womb Healing:* Pain, shame, memories of humiliation, sexual trauma, miscarriages, and relationship wounds all settle deep inside the womb.

Through specific yoga postures, breathwork, and guided womb meditations, these energetic imprints can be released, making the womb a place of love rather than pain.

- *Feminine Awakening & Self-Love:* When a woman reconnects with her femininity—by embracing her cycles, loving her curves, honoring her creative energy—miracles happen in her hormonal and nervous systems.

Self-love is the most powerful hormone regulator known to humankind.

- *Daily Practical Tools:* Healing is not only spiritual. It is deeply **practical**.
    - Morning rituals
    - Journaling
    - Herbal teas
    - Forgiveness exercises
    - Body-mind check-ins
    - Menstrual tracking
    - Nourishing foods

These small tools, used consistently, rewire your biology and psychology.

- *Mindful Relationship with Pain:* Instead of escaping pain, healing invites you to listen to it. Pain is not your enemy. It is a sacred message from your body asking for change.

Painkillers Are Not the Solution—They Are a Mask

Painkillers may provide short-term relief, but long-term damage.

Side Effects of Regular Painkiller Use

- Digestive Issues: Gas, ulcers, indigestion
- Kidney & Liver Toxicity: Organ stress from chemical overload
- Hormonal Disruption: Interrupting the body's natural hormonal rhythm
- Masking Serious Problems: Such as endometriosis, PCOS, or fibroids
- Mental Dependency: Reaching for pills instead of addressing root causes
- Scientific Evidence:
    - Harvard Health reports that NSAIDs block natural inflammation needed for healing.
    - Indian research found 40% of long-term painkiller users experienced hormonal imbalances.
    - AJOG Study: NSAIDs can delay or block ovulation.

Then What is the Alternative?

Become a Body Listener, Not a Pill Popper.

- **Menstrual Healing Tools:**
    - **Menstrual Breathing & Womb Yoga**

Gentle asanas like:

- ✓ Child's Pose (*Balasana*)
- ✓ Butterfly Pose (*Baddha Konasana*)
- ✓ Cat-Cow (*Marjaryasana-Bitilasana*)

Breathwork techniques like:

- ✓ Bhramari Pranayama
- ✓ Ujjayi Breath

These relax the nervous system and reduce menstrual discomfort naturally.

- **Natural Pain Relievers**

Herbs like:

- ✓ *Tulsi* (Holy Basil)
- ✓ Ginger
- ✓ Fennel

- ✓ Mint

Warm herbal teas made from these act as natural anti-inflammatories.

- o **Emotional Journaling:** Write freely: How do you feel before/during your period? Where do you feel tension? What do you wish to express?

This helps release emotional toxins trapped in the womb.

- o **Pain is a Message: "Listen to Me.":** When the body is in pain, it is asking you to change.

Irregular periods, PCOS, infertility, and mood swings are not random. They are rooted in deeper emotional and lifestyle imbalances.

Your Body Wants to be Heard

Start by placing your hands on your womb and say:

I am listening to you. You are safe. You are loved.

Sacred Layers of Menstrual Healing

- **Self-Love Practices**

Look in the mirror and say:

"I am whole. I am perfect. I love myself."

- **Womb Forgiveness Ritual**

Place your hand on your womb and whisper:

"I am sorry. Please forgive me. Thank you. I love you."

- **Womb Breathing**

Close your eyes. Breathe slowly into your belly. Visualize your womb glowing with healing light.

- **Herbal Hormonal Support**

Ayurvedic herbs like Ashoka, Shatavari, and Ghee with warm water help restore hormonal rhythm.

- **Cycle-Balancing Movement**

Practice gentle yoga or pranayama daily to improve blood flow and emotional resilience.

Hormones Understand Emotions

Hormones do not respond only to food or medicine. They respond to how you feel inside.

If you constantly feel overwhelmed, feel you must be perfect, hate your body and feel ashamed of your menstruation, then your hormones also feel lost.

Emotions are the secret directors of your menstrual health.

Reclaim Your Cycle, Reclaim Your Power

Your menstrual cycle is your personal rhythm. Every month, your body offers you a journey of creation, letting go, reflection, and rebirth.

If you can learn to walk this path with awareness, you will find freedom from pain, irregularity, and shame.

You will become whole again. You will become **you** again.

Healing is not a destination. It is a sacred return to your divine rhythm.

Your womb is listening. Are you?

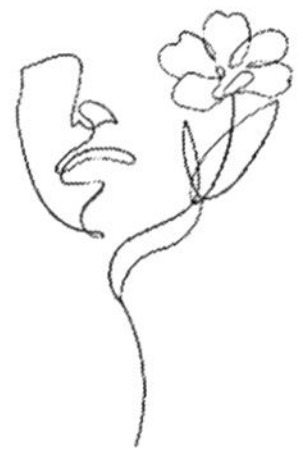

Chapter 8 | Hormones Are Not Just Chemicals: They Are the Voice of Your Emotions

What if someone tells you that the emotional burdens you silently carry in your heart might be the very reason your periods are irregular, painful, or missing altogether?

Hormones are often viewed only as biological substances—as secretions regulated by glands to maintain physical balance. But the deeper truth, often ignored in modern medicine, is this: hormones don't just respond to what we eat or how much we sleep. They respond to what we feel, how we think, and what unresolved emotional stories we are still holding inside.

Hormones are not isolated messengers in the body; they are subtle, intelligent, and deeply attuned to a woman's emotional life.

Emotions Speak in Hormones

Let us explore the invisible bridge between your feelings and your endocrine system. Every single emotion you feel sends ripples across your hormonal harmony.

Hormones Are Not Just Chemicals: They Are the Voice of Your Emotions

Emotion	Hormonal Disruption
Chronic stress, anxiety	↑ Cortisol, ↓ Progesterone
Anger, guilt	Estrogen imbalance
Shame, body hatred	↓ Thyroid hormones
Lack of love, self-hatred	↓ Oxytocin, ↓ Dopamine

Table 8.1

These are not just theoretical connections. Scientific research has proven again and again that long-term emotional distress alters brain chemistry, increases stress hormones, and suppresses reproductive function. That's why emotional healing is not optional—it is essential.

How to Balance Hormones by Healing Emotions

- **Self-Acceptance: The First Hormonal Medicine**

Most women have been taught to criticize themselves.
"I am not beautiful enough."
"I am too emotional."
"I am not as good as others."

These statements do not just remain in the mind; they transmit sadness, stress, and resistance to the body. And over time, they disrupt hormonal balance.

- **Healing Practice**

Every morning, stand in front of a mirror and say to yourself:

✓ I accept myself as I am.

✓ I am complete, just the way I am.

Look into your own eyes. Let your nervous system know that you are finally choosing to love instead of rejecting yourself.

- **Heal the Body and Mind Together**

Hormonal balance is not just emotional. Your body also needs movement, relaxation, and safety.

- **Daily Healing Ritual**:
  - ✓ **20 minutes of gentle yoga**: Focus on poses such as Butterfly (*Baddha Konasana*), Cat-Cow (*Marjaryasana-Bitilasana*), and Seated Forward Fold (*Paschimottanasana*) to support the reproductive system.
  - ✓ **10 minutes of Womb Breathing Meditation**: Close your eyes. Put both hands on your lower belly. Inhale deeply. Imagine your womb as a calm, peaceful place. Exhale all the tension.

This small investment every day creates a massive hormonal transformation over time.

- **Gratitude Journaling: Rewire Your Brain Chemistry**

Your mind constantly records what's missing, what's painful, what can go wrong.

Gratitude helps shift this mental pattern. It calms your stress hormones, uplifts your mood, and boosts serotonin—a key hormone in menstrual health.

- **Healing Practice**:

Every night, write 3 things you are grateful for. Even on your worst day, find something—a breath, a cup of water, a kind smile. Gratitude activates healing.

Ho'oponopono: Speak the Language Your Hormones Understand

The ancient Hawaiian prayer Ho'oponopono is a powerful method to cleanse emotional blocks. Each phrase heals your nervous system and brings peace to your cells.

Speak gently to your womb, your heart, or the part of you that is hurting. Say:

- I'm sorry.
- Please forgive me.
- Thank you.
- I love you.

Do this for a few minutes daily. Let the emotions surface. Let your body receive your care.

The Silent Emotional Wounds We Carry

Every woman has a story she hides in her heart. A story of being silenced, judged, betrayed, touched without consent, left behind, and blamed.

These stories become emotional wounds. They may not bleed, but they shape how we live, how we love, and how we menstruate.

Most Common Origins of Emotional Wounds:

- Childhood neglect or emotional absence
- Lack of love or maternal bonding
- Repeated humiliation or comparison
- Miscarriage or abortion trauma
- Sexual abuse or unwanted touch
- Heartbreak or betrayal by trusted partners

These wounds do not just stay in memory—they live in the womb, in the nervous system, and in the very cells of our reproductive organs.

That's why many women have perfectly normal blood reports and still suffer from:

- Irregular periods
- PCOS/PCOD
- Endometriosis
- Infertility
- Mood swings

The problem is not always physical. It is emotional, spiritual, and energetic.

And the solution is **HEALING**.

Not just once, but as a daily practice of returning to yourself, loving the parts you judged, hugging the parts you hid and listening to the parts you ignored.

This is what heals your hormones. This is what brings back your period. This is what restores your joy.

MenstruSolution is not just a method to fix your period. It is your journey to wholeness, through the science of the body and the intelligence of the soul.

Let each hormone be your guide. Let each emotion be your teacher. Let each wound be your invitation to go deeper into the healing that was always waiting for you.

The body will respond. It always does. Because it never stopped loving you.

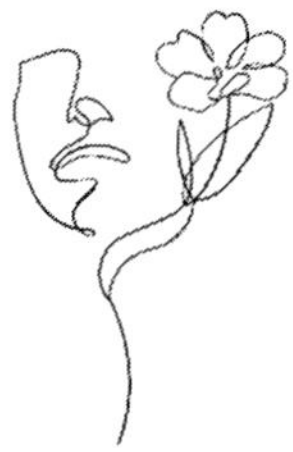

Chapter 9 | We Carry Generational Pain: The Ancestral Wounds in Our Womb

In the sacred circle of womanhood, there exists an unspoken truth: the pain you carry may not be yours alone. Hidden beneath your modern worries, period problems, and fertility struggles lie stories older than you — stories woven into the womb by the hands of your mother, grandmother, and all the women who came before you. This is the truth of generational pain — emotional legacies passed through the womb space from one generation to another.

You Were Born Holding More Than Just Your Own Story

When a woman becomes pregnant with a baby girl, she carries not just the next generation but the seeds of the one after that as well. In the early stages of fetal development, a female fetus begins forming all the eggs (ova) she will ever carry in her lifetime. This means that inside your grandmother's womb, your mother's womb was forming — and inside your mother's womb, your own egg was already present.

Three generations — grandmother, mother, and daughter — are bound together in one sacred moment.

And along with life, emotions also travel. If your grandmother experienced fear, grief, rejection, or trauma during pregnancy or in her life, it could be imprinted in her womb and passed through to your mother and then to you.

The Womb: Not Just a Reproductive Organ

The womb is a multidimensional space. It is a physical, emotional, and energetic center of womanhood. It is the seat of:

- Creation
- Intuition
- Emotional memory
- Feminine power
- Ancestral connection

But when left unhealed, it can also become the graveyard of old pain.

Your womb holds not just your monthly cycles — it holds your heartbreaks, unspoken fears, buried guilt, and the silent traumas that have not found voice.

How Pain, Trauma, and Rejection Store Themselves in the Womb

- **Trauma**

When a woman undergoes any form of trauma — emotional, physical, or sexual — and cannot fully process it, the trauma gets buried deep within. The womb becomes the storage chamber of unexpressed screams and frozen emotions.

Often women say, "It feels heavy here," pointing to the lower belly. That's the womb speaking, trying to be heard.

- **Grief**

Loss — whether of a baby, a partner, a relationship, or a dream — does not always leave with time. Tears that are not shed find residence in the womb.

Such grief often turns into emotional numbness, hormonal imbalance, and a womb that feels cold, closed, or unresponsive.

- **Abuse**

When abuse is unspoken or suppressed, the body does not forget. Especially in cases of sexual trauma, the womb and yoni (vaginal space) contract and guard themselves, creating emotional armor.

This can result in:

- Irregular periods
- Pain during intercourse
- Fertility issues
- Aversion to touch or intimacy

Rejection of the Feminine

Many girls grow up hearing:

- "Why don't you act like a boy?"
- "Being a girl is a burden."
- "You're too emotional."

Such statements cause a woman to reject her own femininity. She may suppress her softness, intuition, creativity — and along with that, the womb energy shuts down.

She may say:

- "I hate my period."
- "Why was I born a girl?"
- "I don't feel like a woman."

These thoughts do not just exist in the mind — they create energetic dissonance in the womb.

Symptoms of Stored Emotional Pain in the Womb

Unhealed ancestral and personal trauma manifests as physical and emotional imbalances, such as:

- Painful or irregular menstruation
- Reproductive disorders like PCOS, endometriosis, fibroids
- Unexplained infertility
- Constant fatigue or pelvic heaviness
- Disconnection from the body and sexuality
- Fear of pregnancy or motherhood
- Recurring relationship issues
- Low self-worth and emotional suppression

Why This Matters in Your Menstrual Healing Journey

If you have tried all the lifestyle changes, medications, and physical healing methods but still feel stuck, perhaps the missing piece is emotional and ancestral healing.

Your body is not just a machine. It is an emotional being. Your womb is a storyteller. Until her stories are heard, true healing remains incomplete.

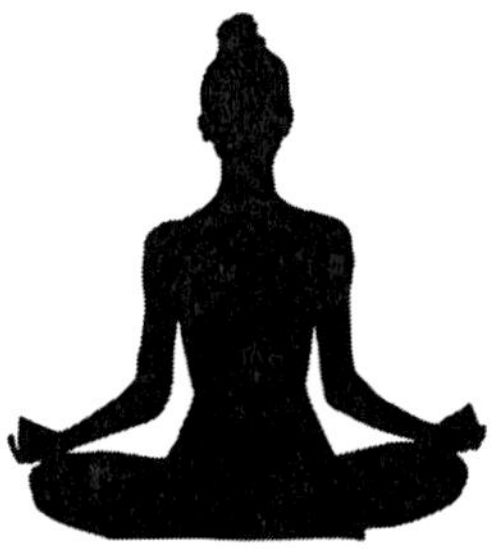

Begin Listening to the Voice of Your Womb

Ask yourself:

- What pain am I carrying that may not be mine?
- What messages has my mother's or grandmother's life taught me about being a woman?
- What do I believe about my womb, my periods, and my fertility?

Gentle Ways to Begin Ancestral Womb Healing

- Womb Dialogue: Place your hand over your womb and whisper: "I see you. I hear you. You are not alone."
- Ho'oponopono to Your Ancestors: Say aloud: "To my mother, grandmother, and all the women before me — I'm sorry. Please forgive me. Thank you. I love you."
- Release through Movement: Practice gentle womb yoga or dance to let your womb feel freedom and fluidity.
- Journaling for Generational Patterns: Write about your female lineage. What traumas, limitations, or strengths

have been passed down? What patterns are you ready to break?

- Herbal Healing: Use herbs like Ashoka, Shatavari, and Red Raspberry Leaf to nurture and relax your womb.

You Are the Healing Point of Your Lineage

The pain did not start with you — but it can end with you.

By healing your womb, you heal generations before you and after you.

You become the turning point, the woman who chooses to listen, to honor, to release — and to rebirth her life from the sacred space within.

This is not just healing. This is liberation.

Let your womb become the sanctuary of peace, not the storehouse of pain. Let your menstruation be a celebration, not a curse.

Let your journey be your lineage's gift of freedom.

You are the healing the world has been waiting for.

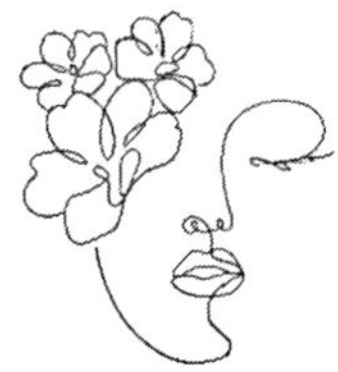

Chapter 10 | The Healing Path: Self-Forgiveness, Ho'oponopono, and Releasing Lineage Wounds

Healing is not a final destination—it is a sacred, lifelong journey back to your authentic self. At the heart of this journey lies forgiveness—not just of others, but of the one who needs it most: **yourself.**

The Art of Self-Forgiveness

Self-forgiveness is the key to emotional freedom. It is the act of lovingly releasing yourself from guilt, shame, and resentment. It means acknowledging your past wounds, missteps, and flaws—and yet offering yourself compassion, grace, and permission to begin anew.

Every woman carries hidden stories of regret: things she wishes she hadn't done, words she wishes she'd spoken, boundaries she failed to uphold. **These memories live in our hearts and, more importantly, in our bodies—especially our wombs.**

When we deny ourselves forgiveness, our energy remains stuck. We cannot flow. We cannot fully bleed, create, or receive. We become emotionally constipated, carrying burdens not meant to be carried for a lifetime.

To forgive yourself is not to forget what happened, but to free yourself from the weight of punishment. It is to understand that you did the best you could with the awareness you had—and now, you are ready to rise.

Ho'oponopono: A Sacred Ritual of Reconciliation

Ho'oponopono is a profound Hawaiian practice of reconciliation and forgiveness, based on the belief that peace begins within.

It teaches that by taking 100% responsibility for everything in your reality—including your pain—you have the power to transform it. You become not just the wounded, but also the healer.

The Transformative Story of Dr. Ihaleakala Hew Len

Dr. Hew Len, a Hawaiian psychologist, brought global attention to Ho'oponopono through a miraculous event. In the 1980s, he worked at the Hawaii State Hospital, a psychiatric unit for criminally insane patients. The hospital was violent, the staff terrified, and patients heavily medicated and locked away.

But Dr. Len did something unheard of: he never saw the patients in person. Instead, he sat in his office, read their files, and repeated the sacred Ho'oponopono phrases: *I'm sorry. Please forgive me. Thank you. I love you.*

He said these words not to the patients, but to their inner wounds—the energetic imprint that existed in his consciousness.

As he continued this practice, patients started to change. Violent inmates became calm. Staff returned to work with joy. Within a few years, the ward shut down—not because of failure, but because the patients had healed.

This story is not just a miracle; it is a reminder: energy responds to love. Pain responds to attention. Healing begins when we stop trying to fix others—and start cleansing our own hearts.

The Four Pillars of Ho'oponopono

- **I'm sorry** — For holding onto pain, judgment, or resistance.
- **Please forgive me** — For any conscious or unconscious part I played in creating suffering.
- **Thank you** — For the lessons, the opportunity to heal, and the grace of growth.
- **I love you** — A deep, unconditional embrace of your inner self, your wounds, your humanity.

Repeat these phrases daily—while looking at yourself in the mirror, or placing your hands over your womb. Let them become your emotional mantra. Let them soften the tight spaces within you.

The Power of Inner Healing

When self-forgiveness and Ho'oponopono are combined, a deep alchemy occurs. You begin to:

- Reclaim lost parts of your identity.
- Let go of the shame buried in your womb.
- Release guilt over past abortions, miscarriages, heartbreaks, or betrayals.
- Feel emotionally lighter, physically freer.

Try this: Sit in a quiet space. Close your eyes. Bring to mind a painful memory, a wound you've carried far too long. Then, gently say:

"I'm sorry for carrying this pain."
"Please forgive me for not knowing better."
"Thank you for the wisdom this wound has brought me."
"I love you. I love myself. I love my life."

Repeat until your heart feels softer, until your womb feels heard.

Healing the Mother Wound

Many women carry unhealed grief from their relationship with their mothers—what is often referred to as the "Mother Wound."

If your mother was emotionally distant, critical, or absent, it may have shaped how you see yourself, how you seek love, and how you parent yourself.

- ***Symptoms of the Mother Wound:***
    - Low self-worth
    - People-pleasing tendencies
    - Fear of rejection or abandonment
    - Inability to set boundaries

- **Healing Practices:**
    - Acknowledge the pain without judgment.
    - Reparent yourself: offer nurturing words, comfort, and protection to your inner child.
    - Write a letter of forgiveness to your mother—even if you never send it.
    - Practice mirror work and affirmations: "I am lovable. I am enough. I am my own safe place."

Healing the Father Wound

The "Father Wound" emerges from absent, abusive, emotionally unavailable, or overly critical fathers. This can impact your sense of self, your trust in men, and your ability to express your needs.

- **Symptoms**
    - Low self-confidence
    - Difficulty trusting authority figures
    - Overcompensating to gain male approval
- **Healing Practices:**
    - Recognize the wound with compassion

- Reclaim your authority: You are your own protector now
- Embrace healthy masculine energy: structured routines, discipline, goal-setting
- Seek out safe, grounded male role models

Lineage Trauma: The Wounds We Inherit

We are the living prayers of our ancestors—and often, the carriers of their unhealed pain.

Lineage or ancestral trauma refers to unresolved emotions and patterns passed down through generations. It can appear as chronic illness, mental health issues, poverty cycles, or repeating emotional themes.

Imagine when your grandmother was pregnant with your mother, and your mother's ovaries were developing inside her—your egg was already forming. That means your grandmother's emotional state left an imprint on you.

- ***Signs of Lineage Trauma***
  - Unexplained fears or anxieties
  - Repeating family patterns (addiction, abuse, infertility)
  - Unspoken grief in the family
  - Feelings of "carrying something" that is not yours

- **Healing Practices**
  - Identify patterns: Journal recurring themes in your maternal and paternal line
  - Ancestral honoring rituals: light a candle, say a prayer, create an altar
  - Family constellations therapy
  - Practice Ho'oponopono for your lineage:

"I'm sorry, ancestors, for the pain passed on through blood and memory."
"Please forgive me for holding onto wounds that aren't mine."
"Thank you for my life and this opportunity to heal."
"I love you. I release you. I bless you."

Reclaiming Your Emotional Sovereignty

To heal is to return to your wholeness. You do not need to wait for permission. You do not need to carry another generation's pain. You can start with your breath, your voice, and your willingness to forgive.

When you forgive yourself, you are not letting yourself off the hook—you are setting yourself free. When you speak Ho'oponopono, you are not denying the pain—you are transforming it into peace.

Let this chapter be your invitation—to sit with your wounds, speak to your womb, and remember:

You are the healer you have been waiting for.
You are the medicine your lineage has longed for.
You are the first woman in your bloodline brave enough to say:
"The pain ends with me."

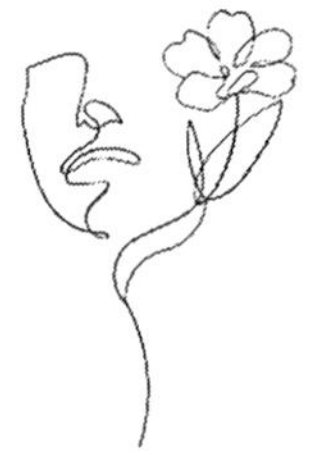

Chapter 11 | What Did Princesses Do During Their Menstrual Cycle? Ancient Wisdom, Royal Rituals & the Sacred Right to Rest

Imagine a time when women were not forced to *"push through"* the pain of their periods, a time when the first sign of menstruation was not hidden with shame, but honored with grace, a time when girls, especially the royal daughters — the princesses — were celebrated, cared for, and given sacred space to connect with themselves during their moon cycles.

This was not just a poetic ideal. Across Vedic India, ancient Egypt, Greece, tribal cultures, and yogic traditions, menstruation was not treated as a monthly inconvenience.
It was honored as a sacred window of transformation —a powerful opportunity for detoxification, rebirth, and inner clarity.

Ritukaksha: The Menstrual Chamber of Royal Women

In royal households, when a princess began her period, she would not be rushed into royal responsibilities or social events. Instead, she was gently guided into a special space called the **Ritukaksha** — a private, peaceful room designed especially for her rest and healing during menstruation.

Far from being an exile, this chamber was a sanctuary. It was often decorated with soft bedding, fragrant flowers, warm lighting, and comforting items — like oil lamps, sacred texts, herbal teas, and prayer beads.

This ancient practice of **resting in seclusion** was not born out of impurity.

It was born out of **reverence for the feminine body** — understanding that menstruation was a time of:

- Physical detoxification
- Emotional release
- Energetic resetting
- Spiritual sensitivity

Women were excused from cooking, temple rituals, sexual relations, and royal duties — **not because they were impure**, but because they were going through a monthly internal pilgrimage—a sacred death and rebirth of the womb.

Self-Care Was Royalty's Right: Ayurvedic Tools Used by Princesses

To manage menstrual discomfort, royal women relied on Ayurvedic rituals rather than modern painkillers. These remedies worked with the body's intelligence, not against it.

- Warm Water Baths: Infused with rose petals, turmeric, or neem to cleanse and calm the body.
- *Abhyanga* (Oil Massage): Using warm sesame oil, sometimes infused with herbs like bala, ashoka, or dashamoola, to relieve cramping and stagnation.
- Herbal Concoctions:
    - Fenugreek (Methi) soaked overnight for reducing bloating and inflammation.
    - Ashoka bark decoction to balance hormonal fluctuations.
    - Hing (asafoetida) in warm water to ease spasms.
    - Tulsi tea to calm the nerves.

These were not just folk remedies — they were part of a **codified healing system** that respected the natural intelligence of the female body.

The Royal Diet: Light, Warm, Nourishing

During their periods, princesses followed a sattvic, healing diet designed to aid digestion and enhance the detox process:

- Khichdi (rice and lentils with ghee and cumin)
- Milk with a pinch of turmeric
- Ghee to lubricate the intestines and womb
- Fenugreek water to reduce pain
- Minimal use of sour foods or chillies

The philosophy was simple: **"If the body is bleeding, do not burden it with heavy, tamasic food. Let it heal with ease."**

Menstruation as a Portal to the Divine

Where modern society sees menstruation as a 'monthly problem', ancient wisdom saw it as a **monthly miracle**.

- The shedding of the uterine lining was not just biological — it was energetic cleansing.
- Women's mood swings were not dismissed — they were understood as signs of deeper emotional release.
- Tiredness was not seen as weakness — it was a call to inwardness and retreat.

The menstrual cycle was viewed as a monthly opportunity for **self-renewal**, much like how the **moon renews itself every 28–29 days**. In fact, most women in natural balance with nature ovulate at the full moon and menstruate at the new moon — a phenomenon still observed in tribal cultures and wilderness dwellers.

This **lunar synchronization** revealed something profound: **The womb is not just a biological organ. It is a lunar temple — a cosmic rhythm keeper.**

Menstruation: A Time for Inner Power, Not Outer Performance

During menstruation, women in ancient times — especially the princesses — were guided to practice:

- *Mauna* (Silence)
- *Dhyana* (Meditation)
- *Svādhyāya* (Self-Inquiry)
- Gratitude and Prayer
- Listening to the body, instead of suppressing it

They refrained from loud conversations, intellectual debates, or spiritual rituals — not because they were banned, but because **menstruation amplified intuition**. The veil between the conscious and subconscious thinned, allowing women to **access visions, wisdom, and clarity** that had eluded them in other phases.

It was not the time for performing outwardly, but for **turning inward** — to reset the nervous system, detoxify the body, and open the portals of creativity and wisdom.

The Truth behind Menstrual Isolation: Not Oppression, But a Gift

Much controversy exists today about the practice of menstrual isolation. Many see it as the patriarchy's way of excluding women.

But historically, this was **a woman's sacred right to rest**.

Imagine being a royal daughter and being told every month: **"Do not serve. Do not cook. Do not be responsible. Just rest, reflect, and rejuvenate."**

What a powerful message that would be to a young girl: **Your body deserves sacred rest. You are worthy of being cared for.**

The intention was never to shame — it was to **protect,** to honor the womb's need for stillness and renewal.

Healing to Conceive: The Ancient Science of Fertility through Menstrual Alignment

The connection between **healthy menstruation and future fertility** was well known in Garbha Vigyan, Ayurveda, and Tantra.

- A painful period meant blocked energies in the lower chakras.
- Irregular cycles indicated an imbalance in the doshas.
- Emotional turmoil during menstruation hinted at **ancestral trauma** held in the womb.

That is why, in ancient households — royal or humble — women were encouraged to:

- Take rest during menstruation
- Avoid sexual activity during bleeding
- Do rituals to release ancestral wounds
- Eat detoxifying foods
- Use herbs and oils to support womb health
- Meditate to align with the cosmic feminine

This is because a **cleansed, rested, and honored womb** was the foundation for conscious conception.

What We Can Learn Today: Reclaiming the Princess Within

In today's fast-paced world, menstruating women are expected to do everything as usual: Cook, clean, work, take exams, attend meetings, care for others — even when their bodies are screaming for rest.

But maybe it's time we ask: **What if I treated my body like a temple? Like royalty? Like a goddess?**

Menstruation is not a weakness.

It is a **superpower** — the body's monthly mechanism to clear out toxins, emotions, karmas, and stories that no longer serve.

We are not meant to suffer through it.

We are meant to **surrender to its sacred rhythm**.

Suggested Practices to Reclaim Your Cycle as Sacred

- Create a **rest ritual** during your period — even if only for a day.
- Use warm oil on your lower belly with a loving touch.
- Drink herbal teas made of tulsi, fenugreek, and shatavari.
- Practice womb breathing, gentle stretches, and journaling.
- Do a fire ceremony or a forgiveness ritual to release emotional burdens.
- Call your period your **"Royal Moon Days"** — and treat yourself accordingly.

Closing Wisdom: When Women Rest, the World Heals

The princesses of ancient times rested not because they were weak, but because they knew that their **true power came from their connection to the womb**.

Menstruation is not just about bleeding; it is about **awakening**.

It is the sacred portal through which **life enters the world** — and it must be honored, revered, and reclaimed.

Let every modern woman remember: **You are a queen. You deserve rest. You deserve reverence.**

And your menstrual cycle is not a curse — it is a **crown.**

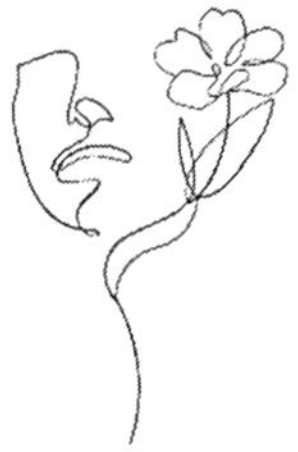

Chapter 12 | Menarche: The Sacred Initiation into Womanhood

The First Flow, a Divine Threshold

Menarche — a girl's first menstruation — is not just a biological milestone; it is a sacred passage, a spiritual initiation into the mysteries of womanhood. In traditional societies and ancient wisdom systems across the world, this moment was honored with reverence, celebration, and profound care.

Today, however, many girls experience this first flow with fear, confusion, or shame. Instead of being welcomed into a new phase of life, they are told to hide, remain silent, or feel impure. This disconnection from the sacredness of menarche is not merely cultural neglect — it has deep psychological and physiological consequences that can affect a woman's relationship with her body for a lifetime.

Let us return to the wisdom of our ancestors. Let us understand menarche through the eyes of Ayurveda, the Upanishads, tribal traditions, and the healing science of celebration.

The True Meaning of Menarche: A Girl Blossoms into a Woman

Menarche signals the unfolding of a girl's reproductive power — the initiation of her monthly inner alchemy. It is her body's first whisper that she holds the creative power of the universe within her womb. Just as the Earth receives the rain and blossoms into fertility, her womb too becomes the sacred soil for potential life.

In ancient Indian traditions, menarche was not seen as "the start of pain" or "burden." It was the awakening of Shakti — the feminine creative force. It marked her alignment with the lunar cycles, the cosmic tides, and the deep rhythms of Mother Nature.

Panchakosha: The Five Sheaths of Being

The Upanishads describe human beings as multidimensional, composed of five layers or koshas — each influencing the girl's experience of menarche.

- Annamaya Kosha – The Physical Body – This layer is formed through food. At menarche, a girl's physical nourishment plays a foundational role. Light, sattvic foods — warm, wholesome, and rich in iron and pranic energy — prepare her body to adjust to the hormonal shifts of her cycle.
- Prāṇamaya Kosha – The Breath and Energy Body – Breath governs energy. Ancient systems encouraged girls to practice gentle prāṇāyāma and deep belly breathing during this time to regulate their energy flow and build emotional resilience.
- Manomaya Kosha – The Emotional and Mental Body – The thoughts she receives at this stage — whether affirming or shaming — become the foundation of her self-image. If her first experience is surrounded by love and sacredness, she learns to honor her body.
- Vijñānamaya Kosha – The Wisdom Body – This sheath is the seat of discernment. Girls must be told the truth — that they are not impure, but immensely powerful.

Menarche is not to be silenced, but to be understood and owned with pride.

- Ānandamaya Kosha – The Bliss Body – At the deepest level, this initiation is spiritual. Menstruation can be a time of divine connection, intuition, and joy if the experience is rooted in love and care.

Celebration is Medicine

Modern science confirms what ancient rituals knew intuitively: **mental health directly influences reproductive health.**

When a girl feels shame, confusion, or rejection during menarche, her hypothalamus-pituitary-ovarian axis can be disrupted — the hormonal rhythm that governs menstruation. This can lead to:

- Irregular cycles
- Hormonal imbalances
- PCOD/PCOS
- Painful or heavy periods

On the other hand, when she is celebrated, supported, and given emotional safety, her hormonal system aligns beautifully, her body trusts the process, and her cycle flows naturally.

Celebrating menarche is not superstition. It is neuroscience.

Ancient Rituals: Science Hidden in Tradition

Let us explore how ancient Indian communities celebrated menarche as a holistic, healing, and sacred rite of passage:

- **Hosige Festival – Karnataka**

In Karnataka, a girl's first menstruation was welcomed with the "Hosige" or "Aarti" ceremony. Lamps were lit, turmeric and sandalwood paste were applied to the girl's forehead, and relatives gathered to bless her new phase.

A "Soppu Hakodu" — a menstrual rest hut — was built with neem, mango, and coconut leaves. These plants are not decorative but medicinal. Neem has antimicrobial, cooling, and immune-supportive properties. The hut became a sanctuary of rest and rejuvenation.

She was given "Ontina Unde" — a medicinal ladoo made from dates, raisins, almonds, ghee, and babul gum. These ingredients:

- Restore lost nutrients
- Support blood formation
- Enhance hormonal balance

This was nutritional therapy wrapped in love.

- **Fruit-Based Ritual Foods – Assam**

In Assam, girls at menarche were given fruits like ripe bananas, papayas, cucumbers, and guavas — all cooling, light, and anti-inflammatory.

This aligns with Ayurveda's "Havishya Anna"—a sattvic, simple diet consumed during sacred times such as fasting, meditation, and menstruation.

The logic? The uterus, like a temple, needs rest. These foods soothe inflammation, aid digestion, and bring inner calm.

Solitude, Not Isolation

Many ancient customs allowed menstruating girls to rest away from household duties. Today, this is misunderstood as exclusion.

But originally, it was sacred solitude — a time for reflection, inner connection, and honoring the self. She was not punished. She was protected from overstimulation, pollution, and stress.

It was her right to rest.

Mental Messages Shape the Womb

When a girl hears: **"You are impure," "Hide it," "Don't tell anyone,"** she begins to fear her own body.

But when she hears: **"You are sacred," "This is your power," "We are proud of you,"** her body blooms with trust. Her hormones, heart, and mind unite in harmony.

A New Memory of Menarche

Imagine a generation of girls who remember their menarche as a festival of self-worth.

Imagine them walking into womanhood knowing:

"I am powerful."
"My body is intelligent."
"My blood is sacred."

This one moment can reshape a lifetime. It is time we reclaim the power of menarche — not just for our daughters, but for the healing of our collective feminine.

Let every first period be a celebration, a ceremony, a sacred song.

Let us write new stories of strength, one flow at a time.

Menarche is not the end of innocence — it is the awakening of divinity.

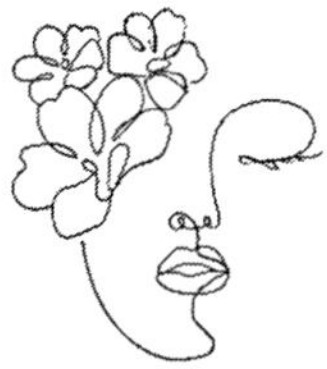

Chapter 13 | Meditation & Menstruation: A Spiritual Parallel

In the vast and sacred landscape of feminine wisdom, menstruation is not a dysfunction or disease to be hidden and tolerated; it is a monthly spiritual retreat, a time for *sadhana.* This chapter reclaims menstruation as a sacred internal *tapasya*—a time when the body, mind, and soul align for purification, release, and rebirth.

Why Is the Same Food Ideal for Both Meditation and Menstruation?

This is because both meditation and menstruation are intense inward journeys. They both:

- Require deep rest and withdrawal from external overstimulation.
- Heighten emotional sensitivity and intuitive perception.
- Demand sattvic (pure), light, nourishing food to maintain balance.

This parallel reminds us: **"Menstruation is not an illness. It's a sacred process of internal alchemy."**

Hence, the diet and lifestyle during this time should support the body's transformative process—not interfere with it.

Food as Medicine, Food as Spiritual Support

In places like Assam and across many parts of India, the traditional menstrual diet includes fruits, moong dal khichdi without salt, ghee, jaggery, and herbal decoctions. These foods were not chosen by chance. They:

- Calm the nervous system.
- Support digestion, which weakens during this phase.
- Nurture the gut-brain connection, now validated by modern neuroscience.

Ancient traditions knew that gut health influences mental clarity. They knew what science was just beginning to articulate: **"Food affects mood, thought, and consciousness."**

Menarche: A Sacred Celebration, Not a Taboo

Menarche, or a girl's first period, is not merely a physical milestone. It is a soul-event, an energetic initiation into womanhood and the power of creation.

Traditionally, across Indian households, menarche was celebrated like a wedding:

- The girl received new clothes, sacred baths, and family blessings.
- Rituals lasted up to 16 days, mirroring the menstrual-to-ovulatory transition.
- She was gifted affirmations, rest, and wisdom about her sacred body.

This initiation was not just a celebration. It was a transformation—telling the girl: **"You are sacred. You are a goddess now."**

Ayurvedic Logic behind Menstrual Rest

Isolation during menstruation, often misunderstood as taboo, was originally a logical practice rooted in **Ayurveda** and **quantum biology**:

- **Immunity is low**: Rest and minimal contact reduce the risk of infections.

- **Electron balance**: Menstruation causes a positive charge to build up in the body.
- **Bathing rituals**: Caregivers bathe to neutralize any energy depletion.
- **Dietary discipline**: Foods that pacify Vata and balance digestion are given.

This was not exclusion; it was sacred protection and energetic alignment.

Menstruation & Electron Exchange: Ancient Ritual Meets Modern Science

Modern quantum biology explains how the body loses electrons during menstruation. A menstruating girl may attract electrons from others, potentially creating an energy imbalance. Ancient rituals ensured:

- She stayed energetically protected
- Others were not depleted
- The environment stayed harmonious

Thus, isolation and bathing were not superstition. They were **electrical hygiene**.

The Sixteen-Day Menarche Celebration: A Journey from Blood to Blossom

Let us journey through the traditional menarche rites:

- **Day 1–3:**
  - Isolation and full rest
  - No salt or curd
  - Khichdi with moong dal and ghee
  - No makeup, nail cutting, or daytime sleep

- **Day 4:**
  - Turmeric bath (cleansing and antimicrobial)
  - Intake of turmeric water (*Pasupta Teertham*)

- **Day 5:**
  - Auspicious bath (*Mangal Snaan*)
  - Re-entry into sacred spaces
- **Day 5–16:**
  - Daily *aarti* by elder women (*Perantam*)
  - Adornment with turmeric, flowers, and bangles
  - Distribution of sweets and tamboolam
  - Song and celebration with sacred music
- **Day 16:**
  - The grand culmination: The girl is seated like a goddess
  - Lavish feast and family celebration

This entire process mirrored the arc of the menstrual cycle: **release, renewal, and resurrection.**

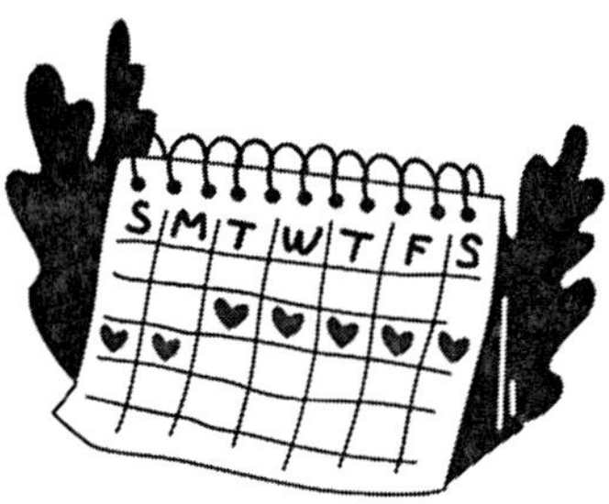

Modern Research Backs Ancient Wisdom

A British Medical Journal study by Zuluaga et al. (Colombian Amazon) confirmed:

- Women who completed full menarche rituals reported significantly **less menstrual pain.**
- Those who partially did the rituals had **moderate pain.**
- Those who skipped them had **high dysmenorrhea.**

This proves that ancient rituals had physiological and emotional impacts.

The Ayurvedic View of Menstruation

According to **Charaka Samhita**, healthy menstruation is marked by:

- Non-sticky (*Nispiccha*) blood
- Pain-free (*Daharti Rahita*) experience
- Five days (*Pancharatra*) duration
- Moderate flow (*Na ati bahu, na aplam*)
- Bright red color like Gunja fruit or lotus dye

Unhealthy signs include foul odor, blackish color, excessive pain or flow—all indicators of **dosha imbalance**.

The Tridosha & Menstrual Cycle

Ayurveda explains the cycle through the lens of **Vata, Pitta, and Kapha.**

Phase	Dominant Dosha	Characteristics
Menstruation	Vata	Elimination, sensitivity, dryness
Ovulation	Pitta	Heat, drive, emotional surge
Luteal Phase	Kapha	Heaviness, bloating, calmness

Table 13.1

Understanding your **prakriti** (constitution) is key to menstrual wellness.

Rajaswala Paricharya: Ancient Guidelines for Sacred Rest

The sacred text **Sushruta Samhita** outlines menstrual lifestyle protocols known as **Rajaswala Paricharya.**

- **Avoid**
    - Sexual activity
    - Excessive talking, laughing, crying
    - Loud noise or emotional drama
    - Applying kajal, cutting nails, or taking massages
    - Daytime naps or heavy work

- **Recommended**
  - Silence and rest
  - Warm, light, oil-free food
  - Warm water baths only after the third day
  - No cosmetics, perfumes, or crowd exposure

These were not restrictions. They were rituals of vital energy conservation and mind-body repair.

The Scientific Logic behind Ancient Rules

- Hormonal shifts affect serotonin and mood.
- Vital energy (*prana*) is being released with blood.
- Digestive fire (*agni*) is weakened.
- Cold or oil can enter open body pores.

Thus, the body's subtle balance needs protection from overstimulation.

What Modern Women Can Learn

You do not have to mimic every ancient ritual literally. But their essence is still relevant:

- Give yourself 3 days of slow living.
- Eat nourishing, Vata-pacifying food.
- Avoid stimulation: phones, parties, excessive work.
- Reflect, write, rest, and honor your body's rhythm.

Final Thought: Menstruation Is a Monthly Meditation

Just as monks enter silence for transformation, women experience this monthly silence through menstruation. Let us restore its honor: **"The womb is not just a reproductive organ. It is the seat of transformation. Every drop of menstrual blood is a verse in the sacred scripture of womanhood."**

When we reclaim menstruation as sacred *sadhana*, we do not just heal our cycles—we awaken a revolution of feminine power, wisdom, and self-respect.

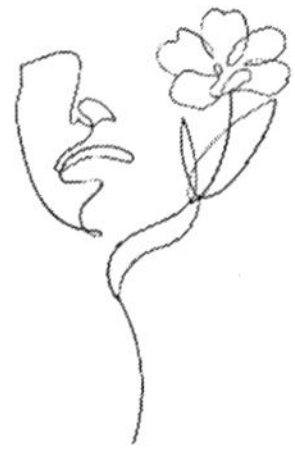

Chapter 14 | Lunar Cycle and the Woman's Menstrual Cycle

A Profound Connection of Spirituality and Reproductive Power

"A woman is like the moon—her body, mind, and emotions wax and wane with the tides of time."

— Ancient Vedic Wisdom

The Moon and the Woman: A Celestial Reflection

Since time immemorial, women have been compared to the moon—not merely as a metaphor of beauty or mood, but because the rhythms of the moon echo profoundly within a woman's physiology. Just as the moon takes approximately 27.32 days to complete its cycle from new to full and back again, the average menstrual cycle also spans around 28 days. This cosmic coincidence is not accidental. It is a spiritual blueprint, a biological harmony embedded in nature's design.

The moon is not just a distant celestial body. In Ayurveda, Tantra, and Jyotish Shastra (Vedic astrology), it is a living symbol of femininity, emotion, fertility, and creativity. The moon governs *Soma*—the cooling, nourishing, intuitive essence in the body—and corresponds directly to *Kapha dosha*, *Ojas*, and the mind.

Women, more than men, are deeply influenced by the moon. Their hormonal tides, emotional states, and even dream cycles often mirror the waxing and waning of lunar phases.

How the Moon Influences Emotions, Hormones, and Reproductive Energy

In *Jyotish*, the moon rules the mind—it is considered "*Manas Karaka*", the significator of mental and emotional faculties. In women, the cyclical nature of estrogen and progesterone echoes the moon's dual energies: waxing (growth, ovulation, and joy) and waning (shedding, introspection, rest).

Each lunar phase has a subtle, yet measurable impact on the female mind-body system:

New Moon (Amavasya)

- The moon is closest to the sun, hence invisible.
- Symbolizes withdrawal, silence, inner cleansing, and surrender.
- Immunity is at its lowest, and *Ojas* (vital energy) is depleted.

Women menstruating during this phase often experience:

- Greater fatigue
- Heightened emotional sensitivity
- A natural urge to isolate or rest

In the Ayurvedic sense, this is the ***apana vayu* phase**—where downward-moving energy facilitates the shedding of the uterine lining. It is a **biological and spiritual detoxification**.

In traditional agrarian societies, farmers **avoid sowing seeds on a new moon**—believing the soil lacks life force. This same principle applies to the womb: menstruation at the new moon is a phase of **fertility potential**, following complete inner cleansing.

Full Moon (Purnima)

- The moon is fully lit and opposite the sun.
- It radiates abundance, clarity, emotional overflow, and peak vitality.

Women ovulating during this time may feel:

- Sexual vibrancy
- Emotional expansiveness
- A deep creative urge

During this phase, the body is most **fertile**, and if sexual intercourse occurs in the **waxing phase** (after menstruation), **conception** typically occurs close to or on the full moon. The **Shakti** energy is heightened, seeking to create, nurture, or express.

The Two Menstrual Archetypes: Red Moon vs White Moon Cycle

- **Red Moon Cycle:** Women who menstruate around the **full moon** and ovulate at the **new moon**.
    - It symbolizes the mystic, healer, shamanic woman.
    - Energy is focused inward—towards spiritual growth, shadow work, and self-renewal.
    - It is often associated with renunciation, inner work, and the path of *Kundalini* awakening.
- **White Moon Cycle:** Women who menstruate around the **new moon** and ovulate around the **full moon**.
    - It represents the nurturer, mother, householder archetype.

- It is aligned with fertility, family, creativity, and manifestation in the outer world.
- This was traditionally seen as the optimal cycle for conception.

Both are sacred, and women may shift between these cycles during various life phases—maidenhood, motherhood, menopause, or during emotional transformations.

Why Menstruating During New Moon Is Considered Healthy

There is **both spiritual and biological logic** behind this ancient belief:

- The new moon encourages withdrawal and rest, which perfectly aligns with the body's natural need to cleanse during menstruation.
- Hormonal patterns and circadian rhythm research suggest that menstruating during the new moon supports a more synchronized endocrine cycle, promoting healthy ovulation and conception mid-cycle.
- In yogic tradition, *Amavasya* is a powerful time for *tapasya* (austerity), *sadhana*, and *mantra siddhi*—thus, menstruation during this phase naturally encourages spiritual detachment and inward reflection.

As **Sri Amritananda Natha Saraswati** once said: *"New moon is the form of Goddess Kali — united with Shiva, where Kundalini energy flows through the Sushumna channel."*

Hence, menstruation during the new moon is not a weakness but a **gateway to spiritual alchemy**.

Menstruation during Full Moon: The Mystical Shamanic Path

On the other hand, when a woman menstruates during the **full moon**, she embodies the **Red Moon Woman**—a phase historically associated with **spiritual teachers, priestesses, and temple initiates**.

Rather than outward fertility, this phase represents:

- Emotional shedding
- Energetic purification
- Deep intuitive downloads
- A time for sacred solitude and healing work

In spiritual terms:

- Full Moon = Peak Lunar Energy
- Menstruation = Letting Go

Thus, the overlap of the two suggests a **cosmic moment of releasing what no longer serves**, making space for powerful inner growth.

It is the **perfect time** for:

- Journaling and moon magic
- Shadow work and trauma release
- Connecting with ancestors and spirit guides
- Awakening *Kundalini Shakti* through meditative silence

Lunar Fertility and the Science of Light

Recent studies in **chronobiology** (the science of biological rhythms) support what our grandmothers intuitively knew:

- Melatonin, the sleep-regulating hormone, is also a key player in reproductive health.
- Moonlight exposure regulates melatonin, which in turn influences GnRH (gonadotropin-releasing hormone)—the master hormone behind menstruation and ovulation.
- Women exposed to natural moonlight cycles often return to a 28-day rhythm, enhancing both mood stability and fertility.

Returning to the Moon: A Call for Rhythmic Living

In today's artificial world of electric lighting, digital schedules, and constant output, women have forgotten their **inner lunar clocks**. Disconnection from the moon is disconnection from the **body's intuitive wisdom**.

Reclaiming lunar awareness can be as simple as:

- Tracking your cycle with the moon phases.
- Sleeping in complete darkness during the new moon.
- Moon bathing during the waxing phase to boost ovulation.
- Honoring rest, retreat, and emotional flow during menstruation.

Conclusion: The Moon is Your Mirror

Your womb is not isolated from the cosmos.

It is a sacred calendar, tuned to the celestial rhythms that govern tides, time, and creation itself.

To know the moon is to know your inner self.

To bleed with awareness is to become a living priestess of the Earth and sky.

Menstruation is not a problem to fix, but a portal of power to reclaim.

So whether you bleed with the new moon or full moon, know this:

"You are the rhythm.
You are the ritual.
You are the moon."

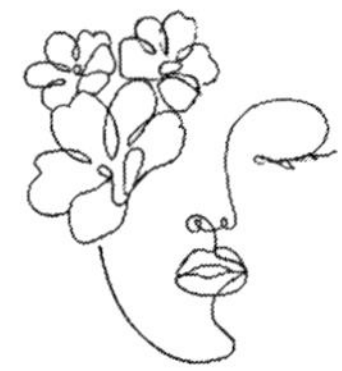

Chapter 15 | The Cycle of Femininity and Ayurvedic Dosha (Bio-Energy)

Understanding the Energetic Landscape of Menstruation through the Wisdom of Ayurveda

"The female body is a sacred vessel, governed not only by blood and biology, but by rhythm, energy, and cosmic intelligence."
— Charaka Samhita

Introduction: Menstruation through the Lens of Ayurveda

In Ayurveda—the world's oldest system of natural healing—the human body is not merely a mechanical structure but an intricate tapestry of **consciousness and energy**. Every thought, emotion, and biological function arises from the dynamic interplay of **three doshas—Vata (air + ether)**, **Pitta (fire + water)**, and **Kapha (earth + water)**.

The **menstrual cycle**, too, is shaped by these bio-energies. Each dosha governs specific functions and regions of the body, and during menstruation, their balance—or imbalance—profoundly affects a woman's physical, emotional, and spiritual well-being.

Dosha (Bio-Energy)	Body Region	Guna (Qualities)	Effect During Menstruation
Vata	Below the navel	Movement, dryness, lightness	Regulates flow, but when aggravated, causes pain and restlessness
Pitta	Abdomen & midsection	Heat, sharpness, transformation	Triggers irritability, anger, and excessive bleeding if out of balance
Kapha	Chest, head, and upper body	Stability, heaviness, lubrication	Leads to lethargy, emotional stagnation, and bloating

Table 15.1: Doshas and Their Influence during Menstruation

Vata Dosha: The Primary Force during Menstruation

Among the three, Vata dosha is the predominant energy during menstruation. Located in the pelvic region, Vata governs movement and elimination, including the downward flow of *Apana Vayu,* the subtype of Vata responsible for menstruation, bowel movements, and childbirth.

When Vata Goes Out of Balance

During menstruation, if Vata is aggravated due to overstimulation—excessive walking, talking, crying, laughing, or emotional stress—it can lead to:

- Abdominal cramps and spasms
- Irregular bleeding
- Anxiety, insomnia, and restlessness
- Cold limbs, headaches, and dry skin

This is why ancient Ayurvedic guidelines recommend a gentle, inward-focused lifestyle during this time.

The Sacred Guidelines of Menstrual Care: *Rajaswala Paricharya*

In Vedic culture, menstruation is referred to as ***"Rajaswala Avastha"***, meaning "a woman in her regal, sacred state." Far from being seen as impure, the menstruating woman was considered in a **heightened energetic and spiritual condition**, requiring **protection, solitude, and rest**. This awareness gave birth to a comprehensive set of guidelines known as ***Rajaswala Paricharya***—a menstrual care code found in ancient texts such as the **Charaka Samhita**, **Sushruta Samhita**, and **Ashtanga Hridaya**.

Purpose of These Guidelines

- To preserve the body's vital force (*Prana* and *Ojas*)
- To balance the *doshas*, especially Vata
- To allow spiritual integration, rest, and renewal

Key Prohibitions during Menstruation (Based on Classical Texts)

These were not meant to oppress, but to protect a woman's subtle energies during a time of natural detoxification and inward movement.

Avoid the Following:

- **Sexual activity:** Depletes *Ojas*, disturbs *Apana Vayu*
- **Overstimulation:** Loud noises, arguments, excess socializing
- **Emotional extremes:** Crying, anger, excessive laughing
- **Heavy work:** Lifting, running, prolonged standing or walking
- **Bathing with cold water:** Invites Vata aggravation; pores are open
- **Massages with oil:** Can penetrate open skin pores and disturb *doshas*
- **Application of cosmetics:** Especially in the eyes, like kajal or eyeliner
- **Cutting nails or hair:** Considered acts of shedding energy

- **Day sleeping:** Increases *Kapha*, causes heaviness

Recommended Practices: What to Do During Menstruation

Instead of seeing menstruation as a disruption, Ayurveda encourages **ritual care and deep listening to the body**. These positive practices align the body, mind, and spirit during this sacred pause.

Do the Following:

- Eat warm, light, soupy meals: Rice, mung dal, boiled vegetables
- Use digestive spices: Cumin, ginger, ajwain, hing (asafoetida)
- Take rest: Reduce physical and mental work
- Wear soft, loose cotton clothes
- Sleep early and rise with the sun
- Maintain silence and introspection
- Sleep on the floor (in ancient times) to stay grounded

The Science behind These Rituals

Modern physiology is beginning to validate what ancient Ayurvedic seers already knew:

- ***Mental Rest and Hormonal Balance***
    - During menstruation, serotonin and dopamine levels fluctuate.
    - Emotional processing is heightened, and the brain is more vulnerable to stress.
    - Silence, solitude, and softness allow better hormonal regulation.
- ***Preserving Prana and Ojas***
    - Menstruation is a loss of energy, not just blood.
    - Physical intimacy and overstimulation deplete *pranic* reserves, weakening immunity and mental clarity.
    - By resting, women retain their inner *Shakti* and recover faster.
- ***Agni and Digestion***

- *Agni* (digestive fire) is naturally weaker during this phase.
- Heavy, fried, or oily foods increase ***Ama*** **(toxins)** and aggravate ***Pitta*** and ***Kapha***.
- **Warm, simple foods** stoke digestion gently and prevent cramps and bloating.

Why Massage and Bathing Were Traditionally Discouraged

Ayurveda holds that during menstruation:

- The skin's *srotas* (microchannels) open wider.
- Oil or water absorption through pores can cause chills or internal dosha imbalances.
- However, in today's world, hygiene is vital. A short warm bath is acceptable—especially with herbal infusions like neem, tulsi, or camphor.

Why Women Were Separated During Menstruation

Though often misunderstood as social discrimination, ***Rajaswala separation*** was a form of reverence. The menstruating woman was believed to be in an **altered energy state**, sensitive to:

- Electromagnetic shifts (now studied in quantum biology)
- Energy exchange through touch
- The emotions of children or the ill, which could affect her recovery

Hence, **reduction of responsibilities**, **time off from household tasks**, and **ritual isolation** served to **empower, not exclude**.

Ayurvedic Menstrual Diet: What to Eat and What to Avoid

- **Recommended Foods:**
    - Rice and green mung dal (*kichari*)
    - Boiled vegetables like bottle gourd, pumpkin, ridge gourd
    - Rice water or kanji for easy hydration

  - Digestive teas: ginger, cumin-fennel tea, ajwain water

- **Avoid These During Menstruation:**
  - Milk or ghee in excess (increases *Kapha* and slows digestion)
  - Tamarind, sour curd, and pickles (increase *Pitta*)
  - Fried, spicy, or heavy foods
  - Refined sugar and caffeine
  - Too much salt (causes bloating)

These dietary rules help **maintain *doshic* harmony**, reduce discomfort, and support the **natural purification process**.

Conclusion: Returning to Rhythmic Living

Rajaswala Paricharya is not a superstition; it is an intuitive science of honoring cyclical wisdom. While the modern woman may not adopt every ancient rule in literal form, the essence remains timeless: ***Menstruation is a sacred time to slow down, restore, reflect, and reconnect.***

It is not an illness, but a monthly spiritual retreat—a return to the womb of silence.

In the dance of *doshas*, in the descent of *Shakti*, in the letting go of blood and memory—there is a deeper rhythm calling every woman home.

Let that rhythm guide you—not just during menstruation, but through your entire cycle of womanhood.

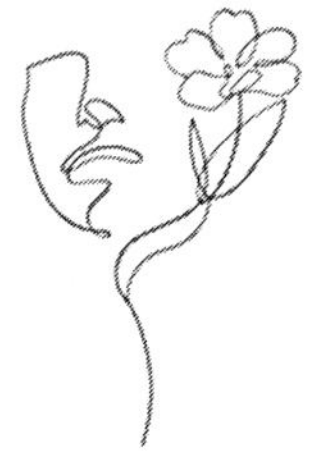

Chapter 16 | The Social and Spiritual Dimensions of Menstruation

Menstruation: A Time for Meditation, Regeneration, and Inner Awakening

Throughout ancient cultures, menstruation was regarded not as a burden, but as a sacred inner retreat. It was understood as a monthly invitation for the woman to turn inward, pause, connect with her intuitive self, and regenerate her vital forces. Today, as modern women navigate a fast-paced world filled with external noise and pressure, there lies immense wisdom in reclaiming this ancestral rhythm.

Menstruation is more than just a biological function. It is a spiritual mirror, a time to reflect, a time to rest, a time to reset.

The ancient Vedic wisdom emphasized the three Rs for menstruating women: **Rest, Restraint, and Regeneration**. This approach is not about oppression or restriction — it is about *deep self-respect*, honoring the body when it speaks the loudest, and nurturing it back to full creative capacity.

The Lunar Connection: Moon and the Menstrual Cycle

A woman is a reflection of the moon. Just as the moon waxes and wanes, influencing tides, plants, and all forms of life, so too does it govern the delicate emotional and hormonal ebb and flow in a woman's body.

The average menstrual cycle is approximately 27.3 days — nearly identical to the moon's lunar cycle. In both *Ayurveda* and *Jyotisha* (Vedic astrology), the moon is revered as the **symbol of the mind and femininity**. This is not metaphorical — it is biological and spiritual truth.

- **New Moon (*Amavasya*)**: When the moon is dark and closest to the sun, many women experience emotional sensitivity, fatigue, and inner chaos. Immunity drops, and *Ojas* (vital energy) is low. This is why menstruation on a new moon is often challenging — but it is also a sign of a *healthy* and fertile cycle.
- **Full Moon (*Purnima*)**: Opposite the Earth, the moon radiates fullness. Women feel more energetic, joyful, and emotionally expansive. Menstruating during this time often indicates that the body is focused on cleansing rather than reproduction.

Lunar Phase	Physical Interpretation	Spiritual Interpretation
Menstruation on New Moon	Body preparing for ovulation and conception	A time of silence, penance, and deep meditation
Menstruation on Full Moon	Less favorable for conception	A time for inner emotional release, intuitive insight

Table 16.1

In Vedic Tantric teachings, *Amavasya* is considered the form of Goddess Kali — a time of inner death and rebirth, of *Kundalini* awakening and surrender. This reinforces the understanding that menstruation is not an impurity but a spiritual reset encoded in a woman's biology.

The Feminine Earth: Mother Nature and the Menstrual Cycle

In Indian tradition, the Earth is not just a planet — she is **Mother Earth (*Dharti Maa*)**. She bleeds, rests, rejuvenates, and creates — just like a woman. The word *Ṛtu* in Sanskrit signifies both seasons and the menstrual cycle, reinforcing this profound correlation.

Just as the body experiences the rise and fall of ***Vata, Pitta, and Kapha*** energies throughout the menstrual phases, Earth also cycles through seasonal *doshic* changes. In Ayurveda, this ancient knowledge is called ***Ṛtucārya*** — the science of seasonal alignment.

Solar Cycle	Period	Impact on Body
Uttarayana (Sun moving North)	Winter to Summer	Absorption increases; energy depletes
Dakshinayana (Sun moving South)	Monsoon to Autumn	Vitality increases; ideal for conception

Table 16.2

In summer — when nature is dry, weak, and unproductive — Mother Earth enters her menstrual phase. This is the basis for festivals like Ambubachi (Assam) and Raja Parba (Odisha), where the Earth is believed to menstruate, and is lovingly allowed to rest.

In South India, couples are advised to abstain during this time, symbolizing respect for nature's cycle.

Autumn (*Hemanta Ritu*), by contrast, is governed by *Kapha dosha* — cool, fertile, and stable — making it an ideal season for conception. It is no coincidence that weddings and pregnancies are often planned during this period in Indian culture.

This intimate mirror between a woman's cycle and nature's rhythm invites us to realize that menstruation is not a monthly illness. It is monthly wisdom.

Ancient Wisdom, Modern Crisis: Emotional Trauma and Hormonal Imbalance

Menstruation does not just respond to biology — it echoes the soul's environment. In today's households, especially where love is replaced by tension, and respect is buried under criticism or emotional absence, girls silently absorb these vibrations.

Studies, traditions, and observations show that parental conflict, emotional neglect, and toxic family environments directly disrupt the emotional safety a girl needs to develop a healthy menstrual and reproductive rhythm.

Effects of Family and Emotional Dysfunction on the Menstrual Cycle:

- Irregular Periods: Emotional stress disrupts the hypothalamic-pituitary-adrenal (HPA) axis, which regulates reproductive hormones. Periods may become erratic, delayed, or prematurely frequent.
- PCOD/PCOS: Prolonged stress increases cortisol, destabilizes insulin and sex hormone levels, causing cystic ovaries, weight gain, and acne.
- Dysmenorrhea (Menstrual Pain): Uterine muscles, tense from unresolved emotional trauma, contract painfully. Girls may be bedridden or incapacitated.
- Depression, Self-Hate, and Suicidal Thoughts: Each cycle brings an emotional purge. If a girl is surrounded by judgment, comparison, or constant criticism, she begins to internalize these feelings, leading to severe emotional crises during her periods.

The Forgotten Culture: When Menstruation Guided Society

There was a time — in indigenous tribes, Vedic villages, and matriarchal cultures — when women's cycles determined the rhythm of collective life. When a woman bled, she was revered as a channel of divine power. Entire communities adjusted their pace, rituals, and rest around her.

The bleeding woman was not isolated as impure. She was *set apart* because she was powerful — more connected to the unseen, to spirit, to life itself.

This wisdom must return. Not for nostalgia, but because the survival of our sanity, sustainability, and sacredness depends on it.

Let the **MenstruSolution** not just teach women how to manage their periods, but how to reclaim them as a sacred rhythm, a spiritual map, and a powerful feminine force.

Because when women bleed consciously, the world heals collectively.

Chapter 17 | The Way Forward: Healing the Womb, Healing the World

In the modern era, with all our progress and information, one essential truth still remains overlooked: a woman's menstrual cycle is not just a bodily function, but a gateway to self-awareness, emotional cleansing, and spiritual power. In a world where femininity is constantly under pressure to conform, compete, and compromise, what is the real solution? How can we restore balance to a woman's inner world and, by extension, to families, communities, and nations?

Let us explore the multidimensional solutions that go beyond medicine and machines — the inner and outer revolutions that need to happen so menstruation can be honored as the sacred flow it truly is.

A Loving Home: The True Beginning of Menstrual Health

Healing begins at home. Before any pill, product, or program, a girl needs a peaceful and loving environment to bloom. Children, especially girls, absorb energy. They do not just hear words; they feel vibrations. If the environment around them is chaotic, abusive, or emotionally unavailable, they internalize that stress, which later reflects in their hormonal, emotional, and menstrual health.

The Foundation:

- Creates a calm, emotionally safe space.
- Encourages honest communication and respect.
- Allows children to witness loving, respectful relationships between adults.

When love and respect thrive between parents, children grow up with a strong sense of self-worth. Their bodies align with that vibration, creating hormonal harmony and menstrual balance.

Teaching Girls to Love Themselves and Their Cycles

From a young age, girls should be taught to understand and celebrate their bodies, feelings, and cycles. Menstruation should not be a hidden embarrassment but a natural, empowering part of growing up.

Teach Her:

- Her body is not a battlefield but a sacred temple.
- Her cycle is not a curse but a compass.
- Her bleeding is not dirty but divine.

Help her see menstruation not just as a biological necessity, but as a time for **rest, reflection, and regeneration.**

Femininity in Crisis: The Reality of Today's Women

Today, women are increasingly disconnected from their inner rhythm. In the chase for career, survival, or societal approval, they have lost touch with their emotional intelligence, intuitive power, and cyclical nature.

Symptoms of Feminine Disconnection:

- Chronic fatigue, anxiety, or depression
- Menstrual irregularities or pain
- Hormonal imbalances like PCOS or endometriosis
- Emotional numbness or instability

When a woman loses harmony within herself, the consequences ripple outward — dimming the emotional light of her home, weakening familial bonds, and draining collective energy.

Why Teaching Self-Defense Alone Isn't Enough

It has become common to enroll girls in karate or martial arts as soon as they begin to mature. While self-defense is a valuable skill, the **intention** behind it must be examined.

Too often, this urge arises from fear: "The world is unsafe." "Girls are weak." "She must protect herself."

These messages, repeated subtly and overtly, form deep-rooted beliefs in a girl's subconscious. They teach her that:

- She is vulnerable.
- The world is threatening.
- She must live in fear and caution.

Subconscious Programming: The Hidden Blueprint

Every child carries within them not only their own experiences but the unresolved fears, traumas, and beliefs of their ancestors. This is now scientifically recognized through **epigenetics** — the study of how trauma and emotional states can be biologically inherited.

When generations of women have lived in fear, silence, or oppression, their descendants inherit those wounds unless conscious healing occurs.

Neuroscience confirms: **The thoughts we think repeatedly create chemical reactions in our brain and body.** If those thoughts are of fear, danger, or weakness, the body lives in fight-or-flight mode, disrupting hormones and menstrual health.

The Power of Thought: You Become What You Believe

Swami Vivekananda's wisdom rings truer than ever: ***"You become what you think. If you think yourself weak, you will be weak. If you think yourself powerful, you will become powerful."***

This is echoed in quantum physics and the **Law of Attraction**. When a girl constantly hears and believes she is unsafe or weak, she begins to emit that vibration—and, unfortunately, life responds to it. This is known as the **self-fulfilling prophecy.**

☞ **Fear attracts fear. Strength attracts strength.**

Understanding the Divine Complementarity of Male & Female Energies

Nature did not create men and women to compete, but to **complement one another.** Each gender carries unique strengths:

- **Men:**
    - Higher testosterone
    - Physical strength
    - Quick response and logical analysis

- **Women:**
    - Higher estrogen & progesterone
    - Emotional intelligence
    - Patience, nurturing, and cyclic intuition

These differences are not flaws. They are part of a divine dance in which each fulfills a role in creation and preservation.

Redefining Motherhood beyond Childbirth

A woman does not become a mother only by giving birth. She becomes a mother the moment she takes responsibility for **nurturing, guiding, protecting, and creating**.

Many women who have never conceived biologically carry the essence of motherhood deeply within them. Conversely, some biological mothers never awaken the consciousness of nurturing.

True motherhood is:

- An emotional power

- A psychological role
- A spiritual vibration

A girl disconnected from her body and emotions may find it difficult to feel or express this power.

The New Paradigm: Empowerment through Awareness

If we want real change, we must raise our daughters with **confidence, consciousness, and courage**. Here are the new mantras:

- "You are not just to be protected; you are capable of protecting others."
- "Your strength comes from your love, not your fear."
- "Being a mother is not a role; it is a power."

Reframing Menstruation: Not Shame, But Sacred

We must reclaim menstruation as a deeply **biological, emotional, and spiritual** process. It is a cycle of creation, a rhythm of the cosmos manifesting within a woman's body.

It is the very basis of life and deserves respect, care, and sacred recognition.

Case Study: The Sabarimala Temple Controversy

In recent years, menstruation has found itself at the heart of heated debates — most notably the Sabarimala controversy.

- **The Ancient Context:** The temple's presiding deity, Lord Ayyappa, is a *Naishtika Brahmachari* — a vow-bound celibate. Traditionally, women between the menstruating ages of 10 to 50 were asked not to enter, not because of impurity, but to honor the celibate vow of the deity.
- **The Modern Misinterpretation:** Media narratives twisted the issue into a debate over menstrual impurity and gender discrimination, ignoring the deeper spiritual symbolism behind the restriction.

☞ **This controversy reveals a deeper need:** We must educate society not only with facts but with emotional and spiritual literacy. Menstruation is not impure. It is misunderstood.

The Final Truth

When women are truly honored for their cycles, when girls are raised to love their womb, when society acknowledges that menstruation is not a defect but a divine rhythm — we will see not only healthier bodies, but a more peaceful, intuitive, and balanced world.

Because when a woman heals, generations heal.
When a mother is empowered, a nation is born anew.
When menstruation is embraced,
the divine feminine awakens.

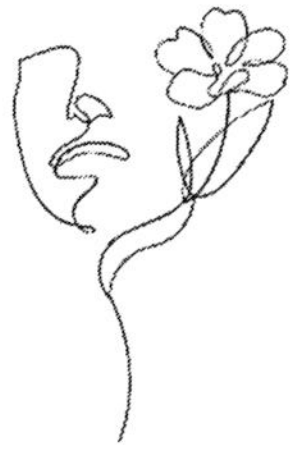

Chapter 18 | Moon & Menstrual Cycle: Ancient Wisdom and the Intrinsic Connection to Women's Life

From the dawn of civilization, cultures around the globe have recognized a mysterious yet profound link between the lunar and menstrual cycles. This is not a coincidence but a cosmic alignment—one that has governed the biological, emotional, and spiritual landscapes of women's lives for millennia.

The very word "menstruation" finds its roots in the Latin word *mensis* (month) and the Greek word *mene* (moon), both signifying the intrinsic rhythmic alignment between the moon and a woman's womb. The etymology itself is a testimony to this ancient, sacred connection. The menstrual cycle—approximately 28 to 29.5 days—is almost identical to the lunar cycle, and this natural synchronization forms the foundation of feminine vitality, fertility, and intuitive wisdom.

Ayurvedic Perspective: The Body's Rhythmic Harmony with Nature

In the timeless science of Ayurveda, menstruation is referred to as ***Artava***— a term derived from *Rtu,* meaning season or cycle. Ayurveda views the human body as a microcosm of the larger cosmos, interwoven with nature's elemental rhythms. Just as nature undergoes seasonal transformation, the woman's body mirrors this cyclic wisdom through the phases of menstruation.

Dr. James G. Bailey notes, "As the moon waxes and wanes, so does the woman's body engage in a dance of death and rebirth." In a state of optimal health, a woman's body often aligns with this celestial clock—menstruation begins around the New Moon, and ovulation peaks during the Full Moon.

The Full Moon symbolizes radiance, receptivity, fertility, and fullness—an ideal time for conception, creation, and external expression.

The New Moon, on the other hand, symbolizes darkness, introspection, rest, and renewal—perfectly in tune with menstruation's call for inner retreat and purification.

Jyotish Insights: Celestial Influence on Menstruation

Vedic Astrology (*Jyotish*), particularly the writings of Varahamihira and Parashara, acknowledge the lunar influence on menstruation. A woman's first period, or *menarche,* that occurs under a specific *tithi* (lunar day), is believed to shape her emotional landscape, energy tendencies, and life path.

This insight is not to be confused with superstition—it is an observation rooted in empirical wisdom passed down over thousands of years. The moon, ruling the mind and emotions in Vedic astrology, cyclically influences a woman's reproductive system and emotional tides.

Kama Shastra: Erotic Energies and Moon's Influence

Ancient texts such as the *Ratiratna, Ratishastra,* and *Anangaranga* delve deeply into the intimate connection between moon phases and women's erotic energy. These scriptures describe how sexual energy moves across the female body differently during the lunar phases.

- In the *Shukla Paksha* (waxing moon), the right side of the woman's body becomes more receptive to desire and touch.

- In the *Krishna Paksha* (waning moon), the left side holds this energy.

Anangaranga even maps a daily flow of desire, starting from the big toe and ascending to the crown, before reversing with the waning phase. This energetic cartography affirms how sensuality in women is not only emotional but cyclic and cosmic.

Moon as a Symbol of Feminine Consciousness

The moon does not merely reflect sunlight; it reflects the essence of feminine consciousness:

- Creativity
- Receptivity
- Emotional intelligence
- Nurturing wisdom

When the moon is full, the feminine energy is expansive, magnetic, and fertile. When it wanes, it retreats into inner sanctity—calling for rest, healing, and introspection. A woman who aligns with this rhythm honors not only her body but her soul's deeper call.

Yogic Understanding: Menstruation as Energy Movement

Yoga, a system rooted in conscious union between the body and soul, views menstruation as a sacred flow of *Prana*—life force energy. Patanjali's Yoga Sutras state: ***Yogas chitta vritti nirodhah. Tada drashtuh svarupe avasthanam. (Yoga is the cessation of the fluctuations of the mind. Then the seer rests in its own true nature.)***

Menstruation is a ***pranic purge***—a natural mechanism for eliminating physical, emotional, and energetic toxins. Especially active during this time is ***Apana Vayu***, the downward-moving energy responsible for elimination, menstruation, and childbirth.

According to Yogic anatomy, five vital energies govern the body:

- ***Prana Vayu*** – inhalation, heart, lungs

- ***Apana Vayu*** – downward flow, elimination, menstruation
- ***Samana Vayu*** – digestion, assimilation
- ***Udana Vayu*** – upward movement, expression, spiritual ascension
- ***Vyana Vayu*** – circulation, movement throughout the body

A healthy menstrual cycle depends on an unobstructed *Apana Vayu.* Any resistance—physical or emotional—can result in imbalances, irregularities, and discomfort.

Ayurvedic Approach: Doshas and Menstrual Health

In Ayurveda, health arises from a balance between the three **Doshas**—***Vata***, ***Pitta***, and ***Kapha***.

During menstruation, ***Vata***, especially ***Apana Vata***, dominates. Its imbalance may lead to:

- Painful periods
- Irregular flow
- Mood swings
- Fatigue

Ayurvedic Lifestyle Recommendations during Menstruation:

- **Diet:** Warm, soupy, sattvic foods that are easy to digest
- **Activity:** Minimal exertion, no heavy lifting or intense exercise
- **Environment:** Calm, low light, soothing music or silence
- **Emotions:** Journaling, meditation, self-compassion, emotional release

This sacred pause is a chance for a woman to align with her inner world, perform *atma-vichara* (self-inquiry), and rejuvenate her nervous system.

Menstruation as Monthly Death and Rebirth

In both Ayurvedic and Yogic philosophies, menstruation is regarded as a **monthly rebirth**. As the uterine lining sheds, so do emotional residues, mental clutter, and energetic burdens. A woman's body prepares itself for a new cycle of creation.

To menstruate is to die a little and be born again.

But instead of celebrating this profound cyclic transformation, modern society often treats menstruation as dirty, shameful, or inconvenient. This detachment from nature's rhythm is at the root of many menstrual disorders and emotional disharmonies.

Reclaiming the Sacred: The Spiritual Power of Menstruation

When a woman menstruates, she is not unclean. She is powerful.

- She is clearing the old to welcome the new.
- She is receiving messages from her body and intuition.
- She is syncing with the cosmos, whispering the language of the moon.

If guided with awareness, the menstrual cycle can become a form of spiritual *sadhana*—a sacred discipline. Women in ancient times used this time to withdraw, fast, meditate, and receive divine insights.

"The body becomes the temple, and menstruation is the sacred fire that cleanses and renews it."

A New Paradigm: Joyful Periods, Joyful Women, Joyful Nations

This book, *MenstruSolution,* is not just a call for scientific clarity on menstruation—it is a soul cry for women to rise in their sacred feminine power.

A mother, who learns to honor her body, her blood, her rest, her rage, and her renewal, gives birth to a new society. She is the first temple her child experiences. If that temple is vibrant, sacred, and lit with awareness, the child—and by extension, the nation—glows in health and wisdom.

Let us return to that ancient, intuitive rhythm.

Let your womb bleed not in pain but in pride. Let your blood carry not shame but sacredness. Let your moonlight guide your life's tides.

May your cycle be a source of strength, your vagina a temple of creation, and your joy the blessing of the entire nation.

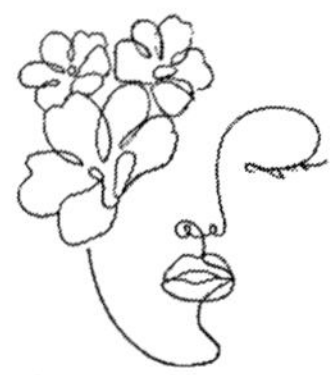

Chapter 19 | The Red Revolution Begins Within: A Sacred Conclusion to MenstruSolution

"When you educate a man, you educate an individual. But when you educate a woman, you educate a generation. And when you heal a woman, you heal the Earth."
— African Proverb, Rewritten for the Womb

We have arrived at the final chapter of ***Womb Matrix: Decoding the Sacred Blueprint of Womanhood*** — not as an end, but as the seed of a new beginning, a beginning that rises from the sacred soil of your womb, from the red river that flows in rhythm with the moon, from the ancient whispers of your foremothers, and from the unspoken grief that you were forced to hide for generations.

The Period Was Never the Problem

Let us say this loud and clear — the period was never impure. It was the perception that was polluted. The womb was never weak. It was the world that was afraid of its power.

The bleeding that society hid in shame is the very source of humanity.

The pain that women were taught to endure silently is the suppressed scream of a planet that has forgotten how to feel.

The silence surrounding menstruation is not just about biology. It is about identity, dignity, freedom, and the right to exist in your full feminine power.

The Journey We Have Walked Together

Through these chapters, we have journeyed across:

- **Ancestral wounds** and **societal shame**
- The **biology and spirituality** of menstruation
- **Holistic healing modalities** — from Ayurveda to Yoga to emotional clearing
- The **moon's rhythm** and the cosmic dance of hormones
- The **law of attraction**, **quantum healing**, and **womb consciousness**
- The need for **a new menstrual culture** rooted in truth, tenderness, and transformation

Each page of this book was not just written in ink — it was written in blood, sweat, tears, and deep reverence for the sacred feminine.

Reclaiming the Womb as the Center of Creation

The womb is not just an organ. It is the throne of creation. It is the original temple — before there were cathedrals, mosques, or mandirs.

Your womb holds the **memory of life and death**, **the power to create or cleanse**, and the **capacity to birth worlds — not just babies**.

When you reconnect with your womb, you don't just heal your periods.

You heal your relationship with your mother.

You heal the karmic debris of generations.

You heal your inner girl who felt unsafe.

You heal your body's cry for rest and recognition.

What We Must Now Unlearn

We must unlearn the centuries of shame.

Unlearn the myth that worth is in productivity, not presence.

Unlearn the belief that to bleed is to be less.

We must remember that:

- **Rest is revolutionary.**
- **Joy is medicine.**
- **Pleasure is sacred.**
- **Bleeding is a monthly rebirth.**

A New Culture of Conscious Menstruation

Imagine a world where:

- Girls are taught to welcome their first period with a **celebration**, not embarrassment.
- Schools educate boys about the **power of the feminine**, not mock it.
- Workplaces provide **period leave**, not punish it.
- Temples embrace the menstruating woman as a **living goddess**, not a polluter.
- A woman can say "I am on my period" with **pride**, not apology.
- This world can be a utopia, but only if **we lead the change from within.**

Your Body Is Not a Battlefield — It Is a Sanctuary

To every woman who ever:

- Apologized for bleeding
- Hid a pad in her sleeve
- Endured pain in silence
- Felt shame for being female
- Was told to sit outside during her period
- Was denied love, prayer, or participation because of a natural cycle

— This book is your revolution, your liberation, your return home.

Your period is not a curse, but **forgetting your sacredness is.**

The Motherline Awakens

You are not just healing yourself.

You are healing your mother, who was never taught to love her body.

You are healing your grandmother, who bled in silence.

You are healing your daughter, who will one day ask, "Is this normal?"

You are healing the Earth, whose seasons and cycles mirror your own.

Every time you honor your cycle, you honor your lineage.

Every time you rest during menstruation, you restore balance in your bloodline.

Every time you speak the truth about your body, you set another woman free.

🌱 The Real *Womb Matrix: Decoding the Sacred Blueprint of Womanhood*

The solution is not a pill, a product, or a policy.

The solution is a **conscious return** to our body's wisdom.

The solution is in how we **raise our girls and boys**, how we **heal our womb wounds**, how we **rewrite our rituals**, and how we **restore reverence** for the menstrual cycle.

Let menstruation not be a problem to solve, but a **power to awaken.**

Let every home be a sanctuary.

Let every woman be her own healer.

Let every girl walk in pride, not in shame.

Let the red revolution begin within.

A Final Invitation

If this book has touched your heart, remember — this is not just a book.

It is a movement.

It is a prayer.

It is a prophecy.

It is the sacred scroll of your own forgotten power.

Share it. Teach it. Live it.

Let the world say: **"She did not just bleed. She blazed a trail."**

In Gratitude

To all the womb-bearers, blood-bleeders, mothers of creation, and soul-sisters — this book is for you.

You are the ***Womb Matrix: Decode the Sacred Blueprint of Womanhood***

You are the medicine.

You are the miracle.

Let the healing begin.

Let the remembering return.

Let the light of your cycle illuminate this world.

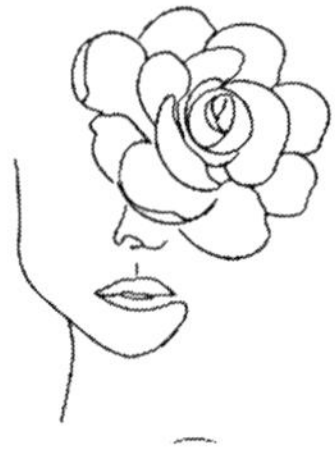

Chapter 20 | Preparing for Divine Motherhood: Inviting Extraordinarily Great Souls as Children

"When a woman consciously prepares her womb, she is not just creating a child; she is creating the future of humanity."
— Ancient Vedic Thought

Introduction: The Sacred Role of the Womb

The womb is not merely a reproductive organ—it is a cosmic portal, a sacred temple where spirit meets matter. Divine Motherhood begins long before conception. It begins in the heart of a woman who chooses to heal, to awaken, and to become a vessel for life with full awareness.

This chapter is a sacred invitation to reclaim the ancient art of *Garbha Sanskar*—the holistic and spiritual preparation for conception that allows a woman to **call forth enlightened souls into her womb**. In this sacred process, the woman is not just becoming a mother—she is becoming a **conscious co-creator of a new humanity**.

Why Prepare the Womb to Invite Great Souls?

In ancient civilizations—from Vedic India to Egyptian temples—women underwent months or even years of preconceptional preparation. It was known that only when a mother's womb was pure, peaceful, and powerful, could she invite souls of exceptional potential: sages, healers, artists, scientists, peace builders.

Science now supports this ancient wisdom. **Epigenetics** shows that the mother's physical and emotional environment deeply affects the genetic expression of her unborn child. Stress, trauma, toxins, and unprocessed emotions in the womb can influence the baby's health, behavior, and life trajectory.

Therefore, **inviting a soul is not an accident**—it is an act of soul-aligned intention.

Signs You Are Ready for Divine Motherhood

- You feel a spiritual longing to nurture, create, and raise a conscious being.
- You are willing to heal old wounds and honor your womb as sacred.
- You see motherhood as a divine responsibility, not just a biological event.
- You are open to inner transformation for the sake of a greater future.

Step-by-Step Path to Prepare the Womb

- **Womb Healing & Emotional Clearing**

Unresolved grief, trauma, or shame stored in the womb space can block the energetic flow of life. Before conception:

  - Do womb meditations and energy work (with a trained guide).
  - Release sexual or ancestral trauma through forgiveness and rituals.
  - Practice Ho'oponopono for the womb: "I'm sorry. Please forgive me. Thank you. I love you."

- **Sacred Nutrition & Detoxification**

Prepare the physical womb as a vibrant, fertile garden:

    - Follow an Ayurvedic or Sattvic diet to balance hormones.
    - Reduce caffeine, plastics, EMF exposure, and processed foods.
    - Include fertility foods such as sesame, dates, ghee, soaked almonds, and shatavari.
    - Fast seasonally or do gentle detoxes to remove *Ama* (toxins).

- **Harmonizing the Menstrual Cycle**

Your cycle is a divine rhythm. Observe it.

    - Track the phases (menstruation, follicular, ovulation, luteal).
    - Use moon syncing to balance your cycle with lunar phases.
    - Celebrate your bleed with reverence—rest, nourish, journal.
    - Heal any disorders (PMS, PCOS, pain) through yoga, herbs, and breathwork.

- **Conscious Relationship with Partner**

The soul entering the womb chooses both parents. Align your energies.

    - Practice sacred intimacy—love-making as a divine act, not stress relief.
    - Share visions for your future child.
    - Cleanse your emotional field together with joint meditations or rituals.
    - Speak affirmations together: *"We are inviting a soul of light. May our union be a blessing for the world."*

Soulful Conception: Rituals to Invite a Great Soul

Garbha Dhyana (Womb Meditation)

Sit in silence. Place your hands on your womb. Visualize a golden light filling your womb-space. Say:

"Dear Soul, if you are ready to come to Earth and walk with love,

I open my womb to receive you in peace, purity, and purpose."

Repeat daily for 21–40 days.

Soul Journaling

Write letters to your future child. Ask:

Who are you? What gifts do you bring? What is your mission?

This builds a telepathic bridge of love and alignment.

Invite during Ovulation Window

On the most fertile day (as per cycle tracking), create a sacred space:

- Light candles, play mantras (like "Om Namo Narayanaya").
- Offer flowers and chant intentions.
- Invoke soul-beings with these words: *"Let only the soul who seeks light, love, and evolution enter my womb. Let this child uplift the world."*

Universal Wisdom on Conscious Conception

"It is the mother's intention that programs the child's destiny."

— *Vedic Garbha Sanskar*

"The body of the child is made from the food, thoughts, and feelings of the mother."

— *Ayurveda*

"Children are not born as blank slates. They are born through the filter of their mother's consciousness."

— *Dr. Bruce Lipton, Epigenetics*

"When women give birth consciously, the Earth is reborn."

— *Mayan Elder Council*

How to Know If a Great Soul Has Entered

These are some common intuitive signs:

- Vivid dreams or visions of a radiant being
- Sudden sense of peace or inner transformation
- A feeling of being "watched over"

- A desire to live more consciously and in alignment

A Message to the Future Mother

You are not just preparing to give birth to a baby.

You are preparing to give birth to a soul who may change the world.

Divine Motherhood is a sacred calling, not to be rushed, feared, or treated casually. Whether you conceive soon, later, or never in the physical—your womb has the power to mother miracles, nurture consciousness, and shape evolution.

Heal your womb.

Honor your blood.

Align with the moon.

Open your heart.

And when the time is ripe,

May the soul of the future walk into your arms, wrapped in light.

So be it.

So be it.

So be it.

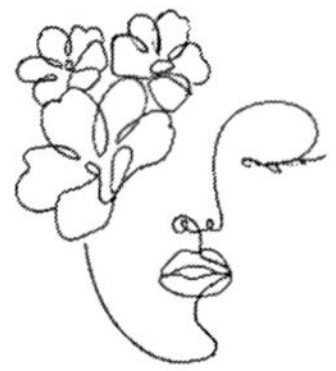

Chapter 21 | Overcome Infertility and Conceive Naturally

A Sacred Journey from Longing to Life
"The womb is not just a place where life begins. It is where love, spirit, and intention meet biology to co-create the future."
— Womb Matrix Wisdom

Introduction: Redefining Infertility with Compassion and Power

Infertility is one of the most emotionally tender experiences a woman or couple can go through. In modern society, it is often reduced to a clinical diagnosis, a silent sorrow, or a source of shame. But in truth, infertility is not a punishment—it is a **sacred pause**.

It is the womb's whisper: **"Heal me. Hear me. Prepare me to hold life in joy, not pain."**

This chapter is not just about medical advice. It is a **reclamation of power**—a return to trusting the wisdom of the body, the timing of the soul, and the creative potential of the Divine Feminine within.

Understanding Infertility Holistically

Infertility is usually defined as the inability to conceive after 12 months of regular, unprotected intercourse. But true healing requires us to go beyond numbers and timelines. We must see **infertility as a multi-dimensional imbalance**, involving:

- **Physical** (hormones, ovulation, uterus health, partner's sperm quality)
- **Emotional** (stress, unresolved trauma, grief from miscarriage or past abortions)
- **Energetic** (blocked womb energy, ancestral imprints, fear-based beliefs)
- **Spiritual** (soul contracts, timing, unawakened feminine power)

Every aspect must be addressed with love and conscious care.

Causes of Infertility: A Womb Matrix Perspective

Dimension	Common Factors	Holistic Insights
Physical	PCOS, endometriosis, fibroids, poor egg/sperm quality	Nourish hormones, reduce inflammation
Emotional	Stress, grief, body shame, fear of motherhood	Emotional release, inner child healing
Energetic	Blocked womb energy, sexual trauma, ancestral karma	Womb healing, forgiveness, cord-cutting
Lifestyle	Poor diet, lack of sleep, toxic exposure	Restore with sleep, sattvic food, detox
Spiritual	Soul of baby not ready, karmic timing, lessons to learn	Prayer, spiritual alignment, surrender

Table 21.1

Step-by-Step Path to Conceive Naturally

- **Womb Healing First, Fertility Later**

Before you invite life into your womb, you must heal your own birth stories, menstrual imbalances, traumas, and womb grief. Try:

- *Womb meditations*
- *Ho'oponopono for the uterus*
- *Energetic cord cutting from past partners*
- *Pelvic breathwork and yoni steam rituals*

- **Balance Your Hormones Naturally**

Your hormones are sacred messengers. Harmonize them with:

- Seed cycling (flax and pumpkin in the follicular phase; sesame and sunflower in the luteal phase)
- Adaptogenic herbs like ashwagandha, shatavari, maca
- Womb-nourishing foods such as beetroot, soaked almonds, moringa, and ghee
- Yoga for fertility: *Supta Baddha Konasana, Viparita Karani, Apana Vayu Mudra*

- **Heal Emotional Wounds**

Unexpressed grief, guilt, fear, or anger can shut down your reproductive energy.

- Do inner child work to release the belief "I'm not ready" or "I'm not worthy."
- Write letters to your womb and forgive her for the pain she has carried.
- Join sacred circles or holistic fertility coaching for emotional alchemy.

- **Live in Alignment with Your Cycle**

Your cycle is the sacred calendar of your body.

- Track ovulation using the Fertility Awareness Method (FAM).
- Sync your life with lunar phases—ovulate with full moon, bleed with new moon.
- Use the fertile window for conscious conception, not mechanical planning.

- **Make Love as a Ritual, Not a Task**

The soul of a baby comes when love is present.

  - Create sacred spaces before intimacy—candles, chanting, flower offerings.
  - Breathe together before union and express your mutual intent: *"We invite a soul of peace, purpose, and light."*
  - Avoid pressure, schedules, and resentment—it constricts womb energy.

- **Connect with the Baby Soul**

Even before conception, the child's soul is around you. You can:

  - Meditate and ask: *"Are you near, my child?"*
  - Keep a dream journal—many women see their baby in dreams before conception.
  - Speak to the soul aloud. Say: *"I am preparing a home of love and health for you. Come when you are ready."*

- **Soul-*Womb Affirmations***

Repeat daily to shift your inner field:

  - *"My womb is ready. I trust divine timing."*
  - *"I am fertile in body, mind, and soul."*
  - *"I forgive the past and welcome new beginnings."*
  - *"I am co-creating life with grace, joy, and surrender."*

- **Scientific *Support* for Holistic Fertility**
  - **Stress Reduction:** Studies show chronic stress can suppress ovulation. Meditation and yoga improve fertility outcomes by up to 30–40%.
  - **Gut and Hormone Health:** 70% of estrogen is regulated via the gut. A clean, probiotic-rich diet supports reproductive health.
  - **Epigenetics:** The emotional and physical environment of the mother before and during conception can alter the baby's DNA expression.

Real Miracles: Stories from the Womb Matrix Community

Across the Womb Matrix healing space, couples from different walks of life—some in their late 30s or early 40s, some labeled with "unexplained infertility," and others with repeated IVF failures—have begun to experience deep, transformative shifts. Many arrive with years of disappointment, emotional fatigue, and physical burnout after trying everything from fertility treatments to hormonal medications. What they often have not tried is this: **listening to the womb**.

And then something beautiful unfolds.

- A woman who had been trying to conceive for over six years finally connected to the grief she had been holding since her teenage years. Within months of working through that emotional release, her cycle normalized—and her pregnancy followed naturally.
- A couple had undergone multiple rounds of failed IUI and IVF. When they joined a healing session focused on womb energy clearing and emotional forgiveness, their connection deepened, stress melted, and conception happened in the most unexpected month—without any medical assistance.
- One woman, told by doctors that her egg reserves were "too low," committed to three months of womb meditations, seed cycling, and self-love rituals. Her next ovulation cycle surprised everyone—not only did she ovulate, but conception followed.

These are not miracles of chance.

They are **miracles of inner alignment**—body, mind, womb, and soul coming into harmony.

When women begin to believe in their womb again, when they treat it not as a faulty organ but as a sacred center of creation, the womb responds. Life listens to love. The soul of the child hears the call.

Even if it takes time, even if the journey is nonlinear, the **shift from despair to hope, from stress to surrender, from infertility to possibility**—that alone is a profound healing.

And this, dear reader, is the womb's truest miracle.

The Soul of the Child You Invite

"Not every child is ordinary. Some children come to uplift generations."

The child your womb is preparing for may be a great artist, healer, philosopher, or visionary. Invite them consciously.

Your womb is not barren. It is **becoming sacred**.

Final Words: You Are Not Alone. You Are Sacred.

Infertility does not mean failure. It is often the womb's call for **healing, realignment, and deep self-love**. Whether you conceive naturally, adopt, or become a spiritual mother, your womb's power remains eternal.

Trust the process. Trust your body.

Miracles are natural when love meets surrender.

"Prepare your womb as you would prepare a temple—for the soul of your child is divine."

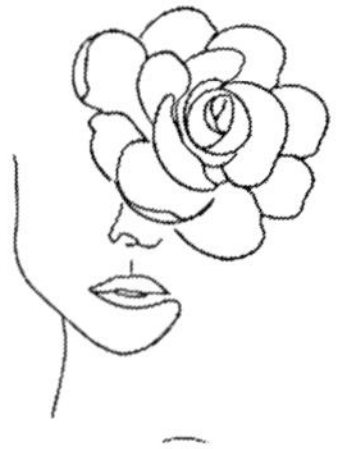

Chapter 22 | The Menopausal Muse: Awakening the Wise Mothers of the World

"There is no force more powerful than a peaceful woman rooted in her own wisdom."

— *Womb Matrix Teachings*

Introduction: The Forgotten Portal of Power

Menopause is not a decline. It is a divine *rebirth.*

It is not the end of youth—it is the *dawn of legacy.*

It is not a biological failure—it is *the gateway to soul leadership.*

In a world that glorifies youth and dismisses aging, we have failed to see that menopause is the threshold into feminine mastery. It is the sacred passage where a woman sheds the cycles of reproduction and steps fully into her archetypal role as the Wise Woman, the Grandmother, the Spiritual Matriarch, and the Guardian of Peace.

Where patriarchy overlooks her, wisdom reclaims her. Where society sidelines her, Nature uplifts her.

Where the world sees "the end of womanhood," the Universe smiles—*because She knows the woman has only just begun.*

Menopause: A Biological Shift or a Sacred Rite?

Medically, menopause is defined as the cessation of menstruation for 12 consecutive months. But in the language of the soul, it is a sacred completion of one cosmic cycle and the emergence of a higher frequency of feminine consciousness.

At this phase, the womb no longer bleeds, but it begins to radiate. She no longer births children, but she now births wisdom, peace, and planetary consciousness.

Hormones shift not to weaken her, but to **liberate her** from the biological urgencies of youth. Her estrogen ebbs not to punish, but to **activate her intuitive, unshakable knowing**—the kind that can see beyond conflict, beyond ego, beyond time.

"Menopause is your initiation into freedom. No longer held by the tides of reproduction, you are now free to mother the world."

— *Dr. Christiane Northrup*

The Grandmother Archetype: Humanity's True Elder

In ancient and indigenous cultures, menopausal women were never discarded. They were revered as council keepers, storytellers, medicine women, and soul guides. Tribes would not make major decisions without consulting the elder women, because they knew—wisdom lives in the wombs that have known both birth and death.

In the Native American tradition, menopausal women were known as "Women of the Wisdom Fire", who carried the flame of prophecy, truth, and healing.

In ancient Vedic and yogic teachings, the *Rajaswala Paricharya* (menstrual wisdom texts) viewed the end of cycles as the beginning of spiritual power. The post-menstrual phase was a return to Brahmacharya—the path of *divine feminine detachment and awakening.*

Across Africa, Latin America, Celtic Europe, and the Himalayas, elders were the ones who *blessed seeds, blessed unions, and blessed the future.* They were considered the living bridges between the Earth and the Divine.

So, how did we forget?

The Global Crisis of Disrespecting the Menopausal Woman

When a society dismisses the wisdom of its elder women:

- It loses its moral compass.
- It repeats wars, pain, and trauma.
- It raises children without vision or grounding.
- It chooses power over peace.

Today, we have universities, AI, and algorithms—but we lack consciousness, compassion, and coherence. Why? It is because the sacred role of the elder woman has been deleted from our systems.

"If we want to create peace in the world, we must begin with the mothers."

— *Thich Nhat Hanh*

And we say—if we want to sustain that peace, we must return to the grandmothers.

The Menopausal Woman: Humanity's Peacekeeper

Violence begins in emotionally starved homes. Addiction begins in unmothered hearts. Terrorism begins in the absence of belonging.

And who can prevent this spiral? The woman who has known the depth of giving, grieving, and forgiving, the woman who has moved through birth and loss, rage and love, the woman whose cycles have ended—but whose soul has ripened into golden wholeness.

She does not act from insecurity. She no longer needs validation. She is unshakable. She is complete. And such a woman can lead humanity back to its soul.

When a peaceful menopausal woman holds a home, she heals three generations. When she leads a school, she births compassionate education. When she holds space in community, she silences violence with her gaze. When she governs a land, war cannot sustain itself.

"The hands that once rocked the cradle now have the power to rock the world into peace."

— Anonymous Elder Matriarch

A Menopausal Manifesto for the World

Let this chapter be a call to action—for global leaders, educators, policy-makers, and visionaries.

We must:

- Restore reverence for elder women in families, schools, and institutions.
- Create menopausal wellness programs that honor not only the physical changes but also the emotional and spiritual awakenings.
- Encourage women post-50 to lead circles, councils, and peace missions.
- Celebrate menopause not as an ending—but as a coronation.
- Rebuild a world that runs not on war, but on womb-wisdom.

Universal Wisdom on the Power of the Post-Menopausal Woman

"The older the woman, the more sacred her words. Listen."

— Maori Proverb

"She is past the age of pleasing—she is now the age of presence."

— Clarrissa Pinkola Estés

"The world will be saved by the Western woman."

— Dalai Lama XIV

But we say—the world will be saved by the awakened woman of all cultures, who has walked through the sacred fire of menopause and emerged as the phoenix mother of humanity.

Rise, Elder Queens

To every woman in her 40s, 50s, 60s and beyond—
You are not invisible.
You are invincible.
You carry the codes of regeneration.
You are the medicine we forgot.
You are the harmony this planet needs.
Let the young look to you.
Let the broken learn from you.
Let the world pause in your presence.
Let the war-makers tremble before your silence.
Because you are the Menopausal Muse,
You are the Matriarch of Peace,
And you are the Womb of the World.

"The blood has stopped, but the wisdom now flows."

— *Womb Matrix Teachings*

The Menopausal Muse: Awakening the Wise Mothers of the World From Bleeding to Blessing — The Sacred Transition

There comes a time in every woman's life when the moon no longer visits her womb with its rhythm of blood and renewal. But contrary to what the world has taught us, this is not an ending—it is an awakening. It is the rise of the wise mother, the keeper of peace, the midwife of future generations, the lighthouse in a world of storms.

Menopause is not decay. It is divine inheritance. It is the moment when a woman's energy, once focused on birthing children, begins to birth visions, wisdom, leadership, and planetary transformation. It is the time when she becomes **a spiritual matriarch of the Earth.**

But here lies the universal truth that modern medicine often forgets:

A healthy menopause begins with a healthy menstrual journey.

A peaceful elderhood flows from a healed womb.

Womb health is the root of a woman's emotional, hormonal, sexual, and spiritual life. If we spend decades suppressing, ignoring, or fearing our period pain, our womb trauma, our emotional shame—then menopause becomes a battleground. But when a woman walks her path of menstruation with self-love, rest, reverence, and womb healing, she crosses into menopause like a queen ascending her throne.

This chapter is an invocation, a mirror, and a celebration.

It brings together the wisdom of ***many extraordinary menopausal women*** *— from ancient seers to modern revolutionaries — who blossomed into their greatest power after their bleeding ceased. Their lives are living proof that menopause is not about retreating; it is about returning — to wisdom, to clarity, to service, to soul.*

And if we, as a global society, honour our menopausal mothers — if we give them space to teach, lead, create, and bless — the world will be a safer, wiser, and more loving place.

"If we are to heal the Earth, we must begin by healing the wombs of her women."

— *Womb Matrix Teachings*

Wisdom & Leadership

Women Who Shaped the World after Menopause

Menopause does not retire a woman. It refines her. History shows us again and again that many of the world's most influential women stepped into **political power, diplomatic strategy, or moral leadership** only after crossing the threshold of menopause.

Below are a few such luminous examples:

- **Indira Gandhi (India):** India's first and only female Prime Minister, Indira Gandhi, returned to power in her mid-50s and led the country through some of its most turbulent times. Known as the "Iron Lady of India," her leadership post-menopause was marked by decisive governance, global diplomacy, and visionary planning.

- **Angela Merkel (Germany):** Chancellor of Germany for 16 years, Merkel became one of the world's most respected leaders post-menopause. With her calm intellect and pragmatic diplomacy, she shaped Europe's destiny, steered Germany through economic and refugee crises, and left office with international reverence.
- ***Margaret Thatcher (UK):*** The "Iron Lady" became Britain's Prime Minister at the age of 54, during post-menopause. She was the first woman to hold that position and ruled with unwavering resolve, transforming Britain's economy and foreign policy through her conservative yet uncompromising leadership.
- **Chandrika Kumaratunga (Sri Lanka):** The first female President of Sri Lanka took office in her 50s. Post-menopause, she negotiated peace talks during the civil war and promoted women's rights, reconciliation, and national unity, drawing on a powerful maternal energy that inspired millions.
- **Golda Meir (Israel):** Serving as Prime Minister in her 70s, Golda Meir remains a global symbol of fierce, compassionate leadership. Her tenure was defined by wisdom, maternal honesty, and strength during wartime and international diplomacy.
- **Ellen Johnson Sirleaf (Liberia):** Africa's first elected female head of state became president at the age of 67. A grandmother and Nobel Peace Prize winner, she led Liberia's post-war recovery, empowering women and restoring democracy with depth and resilience that came from decades of lived experience.

- **Sonia Gandhi (India):** Though she never held official Prime Ministership, Sonia Gandhi's political influence post-menopause defined the Indian National Congress for decades. Her leadership through personal loss, party revival, and international relations showcases the quiet yet profound power of elder women.
- **Zia Mody (India):** A top corporate lawyer in India, Zia Mody continued to break glass ceilings into her 50s and 60s. Her post-menopausal years saw her emerge as a legal icon, a mentor, and a key figure in Indian economic reform and corporate governance.
- **Aung San Suu Kyi (Myanmar):** After decades of imprisonment, Aung San Suu Kyi stepped into global diplomacy in her late 60s. Though her legacy is now controversial, her post-menopausal leadership inspired democratic movements and won her a Nobel Peace Prize for non-violent struggle.
- **Gayatri Chakravorty Spivak (India/Global):** One of the world's foremost post-colonial theorists, Spivak's intellectual contributions deepened after menopause. She brought critical feminist and Marxist analysis to literature, education, and global justice, while mentoring generations of scholars across continents.

These women did not retire after 50. They **re-fired** — with clarity, courage, and conviction.

Healing & Spirituality

Menopausal Women as Healers, Visionaries, and Sacred Guides

As the bleeding ceases, the veil between the seen and unseen begins to lift. Many women across cultures and eras have found their **true calling as healers, mystics, energy workers, and spiritual teachers after menopause**. Their wombs, now free from the cycles of physical fertility, become cosmic chalices for wisdom, guidance, and soul-mothering.

Here are some radiant examples:

- **Louise Hay (USA):** At the age of 58, Louise Hay founded **Hay House Publishing**, which became one of the world's largest self-help publishing platforms. A survivor of abuse and cancer, she taught millions the power of self-love, affirmations, and emotional healing. Her post-menopausal awakening changed the landscape of mind-body medicine forever.
- **Anandamayi Ma (India):** One of the most revered mystics of 20th-century India, Anandamayi Ma's spiritual mission blossomed in her later years. After menopause, she became a living embodiment of divine feminine energy, attracting followers across the globe and offering blessings, silence, and wisdom that transcended religion.
- **Iyanla Vanzant (USA):** An acclaimed spiritual teacher and life coach, Iyanla's global impact skyrocketed in her 50s and 60s. Post-menopause, she launched **"Iyanla: Fix My Life"**, offering powerful healing, forgiveness rituals, and soul interventions that helped families and communities awaken and transform.
- **Maya Tiwari (India/USA):** An Ayurvedic scholar and spiritual teacher, Maya Tiwari's womb was removed due to cancer at a young age, but her feminine essence expanded post-menopause. She founded the **Wise Earth School of Ayurveda** and taught millions how to heal with food, rhythm, and Earth-conscious living.
- **Jaggi Vasudev's Mother, Subramaniam Amma (India):** Known to have walked a deeply spiritual path after midlife, she played a foundational role in the spiritual temperament of her family. Though little is documented, mothers like her represent the silent lineage of awakened feminine wisdom that gives birth to global change through subtle yet profound influence.

- **Dadi Janki (India):** Taking global leadership of the **Brahma Kumaris** in her post-menopausal years, Dadi Janki became one of the world's oldest spiritual leaders, serving until age 104. Her life was a message of silent mind, soul-consciousness, and divine mothering.
- **Clarissa Pinkola Estés (USA):** The author of *Women Who Run with the Wolves*, Dr. Estés's work emerged fully in her mature years. A Jungian psychoanalyst and *cantadora* (storyteller), she uses myths and archetypes to awaken deep feminine instincts and intuition—especially valuable for post-menopausal women reclaiming their sacred fire.
- **Ma Anand Sheela (India/Global):** After intense spiritual and political controversy in her younger life, Sheela spent her post-menopausal years as a caregiver for the elderly and mentally disabled in Switzerland. Her later years reflected resilience, responsibility, and an evolved feminine mission.
- **Gabrielle Roth (USA):** Founder of the **5Rhythms Movement Practice**, Gabrielle brought ecstatic dance, body wisdom, and soul awakening to thousands. Her most powerful work as a movement mystic and creative channel came after menopause, when her energy became deeply intuitive, archetypal, and liberating.

When a woman enters menopause with a healed womb,
She doesn't just age — **she alchemizes.**
She becomes a channel, a priestess, a soul-mother to the world.

Science, Innovation & Medicine
Women Who Revolutionized Knowledge after Menopause

Menopause often marks the beginning of deep contemplation, focus, and resilience. Freed from the hormonal tides of reproduction, many women step into their sharpest analytical powers and pioneering genius—especially in fields traditionally dominated by men: science, technology, medicine, and innovation.

Here are some remarkable examples:

- **Marie Curie (Poland/France):** Although Curie's Nobel Prizes came earlier, her enduring contributions to science—including the founding of the Radium Institute and directing mobile X-ray units during WWI—happened in her later years. Even after menopause, she led groundbreaking research on radioactivity, mentored young women scientists, and defied gendered norms till her death at 66.
- **Jane Goodall (UK):** Famed primatologist and anthropologist, Goodall's global conservation mission expanded after menopause. In her 50s and beyond, she founded the **Jane Goodall Institute**, spoke at global forums, launched Roots & Shoots (a youth initiative), and became an environmental and peace ambassador for generations.
- **Gita Gopinath (India/USA):** The first female Chief Economist at the International Monetary Fund, Gopinath's influence surged in her 50s. Her economic wisdom during the COVID-19 recovery placed her among the top policy-makers globally. She continues to shape financial recovery models and inspire women in economics.
- **Tu Youyou (China):** After years of quiet research, Tu discovered **artemisinin**, a life-saving malaria drug, in her late 40s. She received the Nobel Prize in Medicine at the age of 84, well after menopause. Her success emerged from deep traditional knowledge and resilience, despite being sidelined for decades.
- **Kiran Mazumdar-Shaw (India):** Founder of **Biocon**, Kiran is India's biotech queen. While her entrepreneurial journey began earlier, it was post-50 that she took Biocon global, pioneered low-cost insulin, and became a

role model for Indian women in science and health entrepreneurship.

- **Frances Arnold (USA):** Awarded the Nobel Prize in Chemistry in her 60s, Arnold revolutionized **enzyme engineering** through directed evolution. A fierce advocate for women in STEM, her post-menopausal genius brought green chemistry and sustainable tech closer to reality.
- **Sunita Williams (USA/India):** Though her spaceflight missions happened in her 40s, Sunita's leadership and mentorship roles in NASA expanded as she aged. In her post-menopausal years, she has become a guide, inspiration, and teacher for young women aspiring to explore the stars.

Menopause frees up psychic bandwidth. When the body no longer prepares to create life, the mind begins creating universes.

Arts, Literature & Creative Power

Women Who Painted, Wrote, and Performed with Post-Menopausal Brilliance

Creativity, like wisdom, often deepens with age. Menopause becomes the moment when self-censorship falls away, and creative women finally give birth to their boldest books, artworks, performances, and innovations. Some of the world's most acclaimed writers and artists found their voice **after 50**.

- **Toni Morrison (USA):** Nobel Laureate and literary titan, Morrison wrote her masterpiece, *Beloved,* at the age of 56. Post-menopause, she continued writing novels that explored race, womanhood, and memory with unmatched poetic depth. Her elder years were filled with profound creative output, earning her global reverence.
- **Kamala Das (India):** One of India's most fearless feminist voices, Das wrote bold poetry and prose even after menopause. Her raw reflections on womanhood,

desire, and aging challenged cultural norms and birthed a new language of feminine truth in Indian literature.

- **Isabel Allende (Chile/USA):** After menopause, Allende authored globally loved novels like *The House of the Spirits.* Her later works, including memoirs, explored grief, maturity, and spiritual awakening. In her 60s and 70s, she became one of the most translated Spanish authors in the world.
- **Arundhati Roy (India):** While *The God of Small Things* debuted earlier, Roy's post-menopausal years saw her rise as a **voice of resistance**, a public intellectual, and a fearless advocate of justice. Her essays, activism, and sharp critiques of political systems gained global respect.
- **Bharti Kher (India):** Known for her large-scale bindi-based artworks, Kher's creative explorations matured post-menopause, with mythic installations of feminine form and fractured identity. Her work challenges patriarchal aesthetics and reveres the ancient power of womanhood.
- **Judy Chicago (USA):** Post-menopause, Chicago completed iconic feminist artworks such as *The Dinner Party,* celebrating womanhood throughout history. Her later installations, often meditative and womb-centric, are odes to sacred feminine power reclaimed in elder years.
- **Lata Mangeshkar (India):** Though she began singing in her youth, Lataji's voice only deepened in emotional range over time. Her post-menopausal years saw her as a living goddess of Indian music, inspiring generations and recording over 25,000 songs till her later years.
- **Gauri Ma (India):** A key disciple of Sri Ramakrishna, Gauri Ma became a spiritual writer and educator after menopause. She founded the Saradeswari Ashram for women, blending education and spirituality and

nurturing thousands into self-realized, empowered beings.

The womb may stop bleeding,
But ***it never stops birthing.***
Ideas. Books. Paintings. Movements. Magic.

Social Change, Politics & Philanthropy
Menopausal Women as Global Leaders, Policy Shapers & Nurturers of Humanity

In every era and across every culture, women who have crossed the threshold of menopause have risen as protectors of justice, ethical reformers, and mothers of nations. **Their wombs, once creative spaces of biological life, now become sanctuaries of wisdom, moral clarity, and fearless vision**—shaping families, societies, and even entire nations.

Here are some global luminaries:

- **Angela Merkel (Germany):** Served as Chancellor of Germany from ages 51 to 67, she is often called the "mother of Europe." With wisdom, restraint, and quiet authority, she guided Germany through economic crises, refugee integration, and global diplomacy. Her post-menopausal leadership reshaped modern European history.
- **Indira Gandhi (India):** India's first and only woman Prime Minister, Indira, entered her most powerful political years after menopause. Her resilience during war, leadership in poverty eradication, and bold moves such as the Green Revolution demonstrated a fierce maternal leadership unmatched in the modern Indian political arena.
- **Margaret Thatcher (UK):** Britain's first female Prime Minister, Thatcher governed from her early 50s into her 60s. Known as the "Iron Lady," she brought about major economic reforms, steered Britain through international

conflicts, and shattered the glass ceiling for women in global politics.

- **Gayatri Chakravorty Spivak (India/USA):** A post-structuralist feminist scholar and activist, Spivak's global influence soared post-menopause through groundbreaking work like *Can the Subaltern Speak?* and her tireless advocacy for education in rural India. She redefined post-colonial thought and empowered women in both academic and grassroots contexts.
- **Ellen Johnson Sirleaf (Liberia):** Africa's first elected female president, Sirleaf took office in her 60s and led Liberia through post-war recovery, championing women's rights, peace-building, and education. She became a symbol of democratic resilience and earned the Nobel Peace Prize for her leadership.
- **Vandana Shiva (India):** Though active in youth, Shiva's strongest influence came in later life. A post-menopausal eco-feminist, she has become a fierce guardian of biodiversity, food security, and farmer rights. Her writings and activism are rooted in ancient feminine wisdom and environmental justice.
- **Ela Bhatt (India):** Founder of SEWA (Self-Employed Women's Association), Ela Bhatt dedicated her post-menopausal years to economic empowerment for women in India's informal sector. She uplifted millions through microfinance, labor rights, and collective self-reliance—embodying true maternal activism.
- **Oprah Winfrey (USA):** Though globally famous before, Oprah's deepest contributions to healing, spirituality, and social change expanded after menopause. Her **SuperSoul Sunday**, philanthropic ventures, and schools for girls in South Africa reflect the post-menopausal mission of nurturing humanity.
- **Mother Teresa (India/Albania):** Though she served for decades, Mother Teresa's global recognition and

greatest impact as a humanitarian happened post-menopause. She became a symbol of divine compassion, serving the dying and destitute while receiving the Nobel Peace Prize for her selfless service.

- **Aung San Suu Kyi (Myanmar):** Though her legacy has complexities, Suu Kyi's role in democratic reform and non-violent resistance was shaped during long house arrests, including post-menopausal years. She showed how elder feminine resilience could hold moral ground against military oppression.
- **Sudha Murty (India):** An author, engineer, and philanthropist, Murty's influence grew massively after menopause. Her leadership at Infosys Foundation and educational storytelling have made her a household name. She embodies grace, humility, and maternal philanthropy.
- **Coretta Scott King (USA):** After Martin Luther King Jr.'s assassination, Coretta became a key civil rights leader. Her later years were devoted to **non-violence, peace education**, and the preservation of Dr. King's legacy. She remained a beacon of maternal strength and moral courage in her elderhood.

When men retire, they rest.
When women "retire" at menopause, ***they rise***
As teachers, warriors, peacemakers, and truth-tellers.

The Return of the Menopausal Muse

Across continents and centuries, **menopausal women have quietly shaped the soul of civilization**. From the battlefields of justice to the altars of wisdom, from laboratories to literature, from silent prayers to resounding revolutions—**they are the soul-guides, peace-holders, and wisdom-weavers of humanity.**

And yet, we must remember:

A healthy, conscious, and powerful menopause is not a coincidence—it is the fruit of a healthy womb.

It is a lifelong rhythm of menstruation honored, not shamed.

It is the reward of emotional healing, ancestral release, and **inner joy** practiced over the years.

Let this chapter be a sacred mirror.

Let it remind the world that **the end of menstruation is not the end of womanhood—**

It is the awakening of its highest octave.

Prayer to the Wise Mothers of the World

O Sacred Mothers of Wisdom,
O Keepers of the Flame,
You who have walked through the bleeding moonlight,
And now shine with the golden sun of ripened years—
We bow to you.
We see in your eyes the stories of generations.
We feel in your womb the pulse of forgotten civilizations.
We honor the silence you have held, the wars you have prevented,
The families you have nourished, and the truth you have carried in your bones.
May your voice never again be silenced.
May your silver hair be crowned as threads of ancient light.
May the world sit at your feet—ready to remember what it forgot.
O Wise Women, O Menopausal Muses,
Let your presence calm the raging world.
Let your laughter teach joy, and your stillness teach peace.
Let your hands heal the children of the Earth,
Not just those born of your body,
But all those born of your love.
We call forth a new world guided by your vision.
A world where no girl is ashamed of her blood.

A world where no mother is left without reverence.
A world where no woman forgets—
That she is holy.
That she is whole.
That she is home.
We call upon your wisdom to light the way forward.
We vow to listen to your stories.
We vow to restore your seat at the circle.
We vow to remember that your time is not past—
It is just beginning.
Bless us, O Mothers,
With the strength of the Earth,
With the tenderness of the Moon,
With the roar of Truth,
And the patience of a thousand suns.
You are not old.
You are **original.**
You are not finished.
You are **eternal.**
Let the world rise in your honor. Let the future be shaped by your grace.
Tathastu…
Amen…
Ameen…
So be it…
So be it…
So be it…

A Global Wake-Up Call to All Parents and Educators — Especially in India:
"Beyond Grades: Prioritize Girls' Womb Health for a Healthier Future of Humanity"

In today's hyper-competitive academic landscape, especially across the Indian subcontinent, adolescent girls between classes 9 and 12 are caught in a relentless race, a race to secure higher marks, outperform peers, and conform to outdated standards of "success." But beneath this shining facade of academic pressure lies a silent, festering crisis—a widespread neglect of **girls' reproductive and hormonal health**, particularly issues related to menstruation and Polycystic Ovary Syndrome (PCOS).

- **Alarming Scientific Realities**
  - A recent *meta-analysis* conducted in India revealed that **17.7% of adolescent girls (aged 14–19)** suffer from PCOS—meaning at least **1 in every 5 or 6 teenage girls** is hormonally imbalanced.
  - Among **North Indian college-going girls**, the probable prevalence of PCOS stands at a staggering **25%**—that is, 1 in 4 girls.
  - The risk of **clinical depression** among PCOS-affected Indian teenagers is **three times higher** (36.5%) compared to healthy counterparts (11.9%).
  - Studies from endocrinologists and gynecologists consistently demonstrate a **direct and measurable link** between **academic stress** and **hormonal disorders** such as PCOS and Amenorrhea (missed periods).

As one renowned physician put it:
"The traditional education system in India rarely imparts life wisdom or emotional intelligence. Instead, it teaches how to run faster in a rat race. Girls are being taught how to score, not how to *live*."

— *Dr. A. Mehra, Endocrinologist*

The Domino Effect of Neglect

When menstrual and hormonal imbalances are overlooked or dismissed as "normal teenage issues," the consequences are far-reaching and devastating:

- **Chronic menstrual pain** often leads to the overuse of painkillers and hormonal medication, with long-term side effects like liver damage, insulin resistance, and fertility suppression.

- **Infertility rates among Indian women** in their late 20s and 30s are on the rise. According to AIIMS, nearly **27.5 million couples** in India face infertility—a major portion due to untreated PCOS and lifestyle-related hormonal issues.
- **Mental burnout**, **low self-esteem**, and **body shame** arise when girls feel broken or different, simply because their periods are painful or irregular.

All this begins in the formative teenage years. A small neglect today becomes a catastrophic health crisis tomorrow.

□ Reclaiming Joy, Health & Wholeness is Possible — If We Act Now

We invite all parents, educators, and school administrators to **redefine what true education looks like**. A truly educated society is one where girls are thriving—not just academically, but **emotionally, physically, hormonally, and spiritually**.

Here are **three actionable, research-backed strategies** to bring about this transformation:

Awareness & Education First

Make menstrual health and hormonal literacy a mandatory part of parenting and schooling.

- Teach young girls and their caregivers to recognize early signs of PCOS: irregular periods, acne, sudden weight gain, facial hair, anxiety, and fatigue.
- Share knowledge about **period-positive nutrition**—rich in iron, omega-3s, protein, and magnesium.

According to the American College of Obstetricians and Gynecologists (ACOG), early education on menstrual health reduces anxiety and improves self-care practices in girls by 60%.

Mental Health Support & Academic Flexibility

Create safe, pressure-free educational environments where academic excellence coexists with emotional resilience.

Facilitate **"Stress-Free Study Sessions"** or quiet mindfulness corners in schools to combat exam anxiety.

- Encourage counseling, journaling, creative expression, and support groups for girls with hormonal challenges.
- The WHO reports that *over 70% of adolescent health issues are directly linked to unmanaged stress.*

Lifestyle Medicine: Movement, Sleep & Balance

A healthy lifestyle is not optional—it is essential.

Ensure every girl gets **30–60 minutes of movement daily**—dance, yoga, sports, walking. Promote **whole-food diets,** clean hydration, and **7–8 hours of quality sleep** every night.

Keep digital device usage in check to prevent circadian rhythm disruption.

Harvard Medical School affirms that a balanced lifestyle improves reproductive health markers in teens by more than 50% over a 6-month period.

Womb Health = Human Health

Let us remember:

A girl's womb is not just a reproductive organ—it is a sacred centre of vitality, creativity, and life force.

When her cycle is nurtured, her future blossoms; when her hormones are in harmony, her mind becomes powerful.

And when her womb is respected, **the health of entire generations is uplifted**.

As womb wisdom teachers and holistic healers, we believe: **"The quality of a girl's teenage years directly determines the health of her motherhood, her fertility, and her sense of inner power."**

Final Appeal: Dear Parents and Teachers

We are not saying academics do not matter. We are saying **marks alone do not define success**.

Let your daughter be healthy and brilliant. Let her body feel safe. Let her emotions be honoured. Let her womb be empowered.

Say YES to a future where:

- Girls bleed without shame.
- They learn without fear.
- They live with joy, purpose, and balance.
- Periods are celebrated, not silenced.
- Every girl grows up proud of her body.
- Mothers teach daughters the wisdom of their womb.
- Hormonal health is honored, not pathologized.
- Rest is seen as sacred, not weakness.
- Girls dance with the rhythms of the moon.
- Schools respect the cycle, not suppress it.
- Women rise—not despite their wombs, but through them.
- Fertility is nurtured with love, not fear.
- Every pain is listened to, not dismissed.
- Womb healing becomes a birthright, not a luxury.
- The Divine Feminine is awakened in every home.
- Self-care becomes sacred activism.
- Men understand and support the cycle of life.
- The menstrual cycle is taught as a life skill, not a taboo.
- Women reclaim their intuition and inner voice.
- Society makes space for flow—not just productivity.
- Period products are healthy, accessible, and sustainable.
- No woman is punished for her biology—ever again.
- Menstrual wisdom becomes a pillar of leadership.
- Menopause is honored as a gateway to spiritual power.
- Girls see menstruation as a gift, not a curse.

- Families heal when wombs heal.
- The Earth flourishes when women flourish.
- The womb is not a mystery—it is a mirror of the universe.

Let education evolve—from pressure to presence, from performance to personhood.

Because **health is the real success!**

A Heartfelt Note of Gratitude and Love

"Being part of the 5-Day Healing in 7 Days journey from the last 6 months, curated by Katha Chakroborty, has been extremely transformative. As a woman, as a coach, and as a seeker of healing, I found this space to be a sacred pause — where I could meet myself more deeply, more honestly.

The gentle rhythm of the sessions, the soulful sharing among women, and the sacred container Katha held so gracefully created a powerful mirror for reconnecting with my inner world. My relationship with myself has deepened — not through effort, but through presence, through giving myself time, love, and silence.

This wasn't just a healing event — it was a return to self, a moment of stillness in the drudgery of everyday life. The consistency and safety of the space helped me shed layers of old pain and find joy in simply being.

Katha, your energy, clarity, and presence are magnetic and healing. Thank you for creating this sanctuary for women to come together, heal each other, and rise.

I look forward to walking more paths with you, side by side, in healing and sisterhood.

To every woman reading this — gift yourself this experience. You deserve to come home to yourself."

Amrita Datta, Teacher
Energy & Balanced Life Coach
Health & Somatic Practitioner

***

"Attending Katha Ma'am's healing classes has been life-changing.

At the end of a tiring day, her voice — especially when she lovingly recites 'I'm sorry, please forgive me, thank you, I love you' — melts away all my stress.

These classes are a treasure of wisdom and love.

We learn about Menstrual Education, Gratitude, Womb Healing, and Ho'oponopono.

From Sir, we receive gifts like Akashic Healing and Inner Child Meditation, which have helped me release anxiety and sadness I never knew I was carrying.

Through this journey, I've:

- Understood my menstrual phases
- Learned how to deal with PCOD, period pain, and emotional ups and downs
- Started practicing daily gratitude from the heart
- Awakened my forgotten talents in the magical space of *Princesses' Paradise*
- Found deep healing in my relationships

Thank you, Ma'am and Sir, for creating this sanctuary of healing."

Soma Pramanik, Teacher
Ghatal, West Bengal

***

"This healing journey has made me a better version of myself.
I have learned two of life's most powerful lessons: **Self-Love and Forgiveness**.

Now, I understand my body, listen to my mind, and treat myself with respect. I also feel more attuned to the needs of those around me. Healing brings clarity. It brings light.

Thank you, Katha. Thank you, Sir. Forever grateful."

Jayasree Nandi, Teacher
Howrah, West Bengal

***

"As someone with fibroids and fibrocystic conditions, the womb healing session was an awakening.

The breathwork, visualization, and energy guidance created a profound shift. For the first time, I felt warmth, flow, and softness in areas of long-held pain. The golden light I visualized bathing my womb and breasts felt like a blessing from within. My relationship with my body changed — from frustration to compassion.

This session gave me a new level of reverence for my body's wisdom. Thank you, Katha Ma'am — this was not just a healing session, it was a homecoming."

Priyanka Lahiri, Teacher
Coochbehar

***

"From anger and hurt to understanding and calm — that's how I'd sum up my transformation.

Now, I don't break down when problems arise. I look for solutions.

I've learned to forgive and to live joyfully, in my own way.

Thank you for showing me this path."

Chandrasree Chatterjee, College Student
Srirampur, Hooghly

***

"I joined with curiosity. I stayed because I found healing.

I discovered self-love, acceptance, and gratitude.

The daily mirror work revealed wounds I didn't know existed.

Ho'oponopono has helped me forgive, and *Princesses' Paradise* reminded me that I am worthy of joy.

Now, I no longer fear menstruation.
I celebrate it — with knowledge, positivity, and peace.
Thank you, Ma'am and Sir. Thank you, Universe."

Parboti Roy, Homemaker
Alipurduar

***

"I joined before Durga Puja 2024.
Back then, I didn't know the power of self-love and gratitude.
Today, I do.
Now, I know that hurting others or myself solves nothing.
Loving myself is the beginning of everything good.
Thank you, Katha. I love you."

Minakhshi Dey Raha, Homemaker
Durgapur

***

"These sessions have helped me rediscover my worth.
I feel lighter, more confident, and more grounded.
I now believe — I am extraordinary. I am complete.
Thank you, Katha. Thank you, Sir."

Banasree Jana, Homemaker
Contai, West Bengal

***

"My periods were irregular and painful. I had fibroids. But after working with Katha Ma'am 1:1, everything changed.

Pain disappeared. Periods became regular. Fibroids reduced.

Even now, Ma'am is always there when I need her.

It's not just a coach-client relationship — it's a heart connection.

I love you, Ma'am. Thank you for being in my life."

Sangita Bera, Teacher
Midnapur, West Bengal

***

"A Mother's Gratitude from the Heart.

I came seeking help for my daughter's menstrual issue. She used to suffer from **unbearable pain during her periods**, and despite trying every possible treatment, **nothing brought lasting relief**. Day by day, her condition worsened, and as a mother, I felt helpless watching her suffer.

At that time, one of my husband's colleagues told us about Katha Ma'am and Matindra Sir."

Pallabi Ghorai, Homemaker
Ghatal, West Bengal

***

"Honestly, we were skeptical about healing at first—how could something beyond medicine help where medicine failed?

But then…

What unfolded was a ripple of transformation — for her, for me, and for our whole family, **the miracles began.**

Within just a few sessions, we witnessed visible changes—less pain, more emotional stability, and a new sense of hope in my daughter's eyes.

This healing class has been **a divine blessing** for our family.

I will **cherish this experience for the rest of my life**."

Anonymous

***

"As a thyroid patient, I struggled with delayed and painful periods. But after the 1:1 session with Katha Ma'am, my cycles became timely — and surprisingly enjoyable.

Now my daughter is also part of this journey. I believe every woman should experience this — to reclaim menstruation as something beautiful."

Hasina Khatun, Govt. Service
Coochbehar, West Bengal

***

"I joined because of irregular cycles and emotional ups and downs. But what I found was much more — a journey of self-discovery. Today, I feel balanced in body and mind.
Thank you, Katha, for helping me glow — from within."

Bandana Mondal, Homemaker
Khatra, West Bengal

***

Each of these voices is a living testament to what's possible when we reclaim our feminine power through holistic womb healing. These are not just success stories — they are soul awakenings.

When one woman heals, the world heals with her!

Acknowledgment & Gratitude

With our hearts full of reverence, we offer our deepest gratitude to the **Supreme Creator**—the Source of all life, all wisdom, and all possibilities. It is by Divine Will that we have been brought together on this sacred path of healing, purpose, and awakening. Every word in this book is a humble offering to that Infinite Consciousness.

We express our sincere thanks to our **beloved parents**, whose unconditional love, sacrifice, and blessings have been the first teachers of our lives. It is through their divine wombs that we came to Earth, and through their hearts that we learned the values that guide us even today.

To our **teachers**, from childhood to this moment—thank you for instilling in us the power of knowledge, courage, and truth. Your teachings have laid the sacred foundation of our mission.

Katha Chakraborty offers her **soul-deep gratitude** to her mentor, **Matindra Chandra Debnath Sir**, whose vision and healing touched her life in 2021 at EagleGanj. During a moment of deep menstrual pain, he didn't just act as a teacher, but as a guardian. His care, healing, and divine guidance gave birth to a vision—the seed of *MenstruSolution.*

Matindra Debnath, in turn, bows to the Divine Feminine Power within every woman. This book is a tribute to all women—the creators, healers, and nurturers of humanity. He also offers gratitude to Katha, whose courage and clarity of purpose have given this book its wings.

Together, we offer **boundless thanks** to the **Princess Paradise Community**—a sacred sisterhood of seekers and healers. Your daily presence, trust, and participation are not only the lifeblood of this mission but the reason this book was born.

This book is not just ours—it belongs to **every woman, every family, every being** who seeks healing, understanding, and conscious living.

The day every girl lives her life in **Sat-Chit-Ananda**—Truth, Consciousness, and Bliss—we will consider this journey fulfilled.

With sincere acknowledgement and deep gratitude,
Matindra Chandra Debnath & Katha Chakraborty

Awaken Your Spirit. Transform the World.

Welcome to the **Transcendental Eagle Rebirth Retreat (Signature Spiritual Retreat facilitated by Matindra Debnath)**—a soul-stirring sanctuary where the ordinary dissolves and the extraordinary begins. Here, inner peace is not a distant dream but a lived reality. Step into sacred stillness, experience ancient rituals, guided meditative journeys, and the healing embrace of spiritual kinship. Every moment is designed to ignite your highest joy, abundance, success, and harmonious relationships.

Rooted in the eternal truth of **VASUDHAIVA KUTUMBAKAM**—"The whole world is one family"—we honor a divine vision:

We are not merely individuals; we are radiant souls. And every other human being is our sacred brother or sister.

This is more than a retreat. It is a **global awakening**, a **sacred movement**—a conscious call to return home to your true Self, and in doing so, uplift humanity.

Here, we co-create **Heaven on Earth**—a sanctuary for your soul, your family, and for every child born into this planet.

A world where every being lives "Happily Ever Now…"
Together, let us rise as the **Eagles of Consciousness**—wide-winged, wise, and unwavering.

Together, let us fly beyond borders, beliefs, and illusions—into the sky of Oneness.

Through our **teachings, coaching, training, mentoring, and transformational books**, we are not just changing lives—we are **awakening the Collective Consciousness of Humanity**.

This is our sacred mission.
This is our timeless invitation.
Let us walk hand in hand—**billions united as One Family**—to build a luminous Earth rooted in compassion, truth, joy, and transcendence.

🌍 **Heaven is not a place we go. It is a world we create—together.**

Will you rise with us?

✿ *Katha Chakraborty's Holistic Coaching Services*

→📱WhatsApp: 9932143011 to begin your healing journey today!

---

1. **Womb Healing**
   – Gentle energy work and guided rituals to release emotional blocks and awaken feminine power through the sacred womb space.

2. **Menstrual Education**
   – Coaching on cycle awareness, self-care, and hormonal balance for a healthier, empowered period experience.

3. **Healing Menstrual Problems**
   – Natural solutions for cramps, irregular periods, PMS, and emotional pain through holistic therapies and mindset tools.

4. **Fertility & Natural Conception Support** *(with Matindra Debnath)*
   – Womb-based energy work, lifestyle shifts, and fertility rituals to assist in conscious, natural conception.

5. **Life Coaching & Holistic Healing**
   – Deep inner work, forgiveness, meditation, and emotional healing to live with clarity, joy, and balance.

   Princess Paradise Sisterhood *(with Matindra Debnath)*
   – Soulful women's circles offering love, growth, and sacred support in a nurturing community.